EMPOWERED BIRTH

A guide to natural childbirth without fear

GABRIELLE TARGETT

Published by Gabrielle Targett
Perth, WA
Email: info@alabouroflove.com.au First published 2005

Second Edition 2022

This book is copyright. Apart from any fair dealing for the purposes of private study, research, or review, as permitted under the Copyright Act, no part may be reproduced by any process without written permission from the author.

Copyright: © Gabrielle Targett2022

Cover photograph © photo library

National Library of Australia Cataloguing-in-publication data

Targett, Gabrielle E, 1969- .
EMPOWERED BIRTH: a guide to natural childbirth without fear

ISBN 978-0-97581821

Targett, Gabrielle E, 1969- .
A Labour of Love: an Australian guide to natural childbirth.

Bibliography.
ISBN 1 921064 59 5

Targett, Gabrielle E, 1969- .
BIRTH YOUR WAY: empowering through knowledge to create the birth you want and desire

Bibliography.
ISBN 978-0-9757818-1-4

1. Natural childbirth - Australia.
2. Childbirth at home - Australia.
3. Doulas - Australia. I. Title.

618.450994

To my three beautiful adult children, Jaeosha, Ben and Jarrad who came into this world in the most peaceful loving way. I love you with all my heart and soul and could not imagine my life without each of you in it. I have loved watching you grow into the beautiful adults that you have become. Thank you for teaching me so many of the lessons of life though our journey together. Bring on the Grand babies.

I dedicate this book to all the wonderful women and their partners who I have had the privilege of working with for 28 years during pregnancy, labour, birth and beyond. You have taught me more than you will ever know, enabling me to write this book based on what I have observed and learnt over the years.

I am humbled and honored to be a part of something so incredible and continue to do so to this day.

Thank you - Love Your Way Always

About The Author

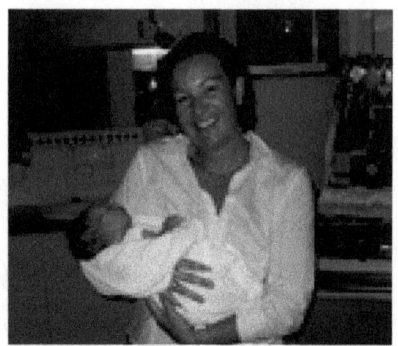

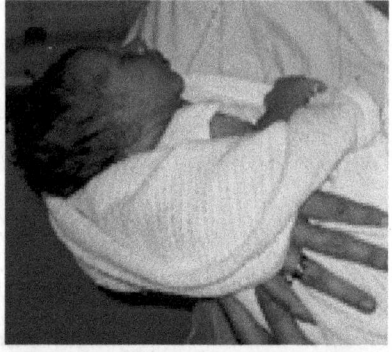

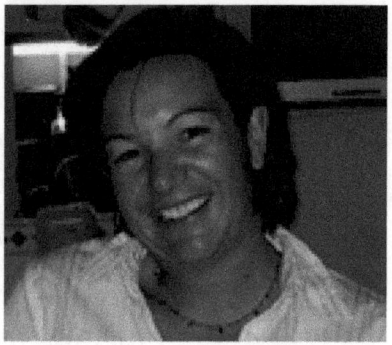

Gabrielle Targett has a degree in Physical Education and has been a qualified Fitness Leader for the last 30 years, specialising in aqua-fitness instruction in the ante-natal and post-natal area. As well as teaching, she has presented many workshops and courses in aqua-fitness instruction and has been an assessor/examiner in the fitness industry for the past eight years. Her outstanding ability to speak publicly with honesty, humor and passion came from her many years of lecturing at TAFE in Health and fitness.

Her greatest achievement came when she gave birth to three beautiful water babies in 1995, 1997 and 1999. After the birth of her son in 1997, she was first asked to attend a birth as a support person. It was at this time she fell in love with the idea of supporting a woman during birth. It wasn't until ten births and three years later that she realised the importance of the work she was doing as a doula (birth support person) and the impact it had on women and their birthing outcomes. It was at that point that she decided to document the births and write the first book from her experiences.

In addition, Gaby decided to train as a childbirth educator. Gaby found that during her aqua natal deep-water running classes the exercise became secondary to the childbirth education she was providing during the one-hour session. So great was the need for education that Gaby decided to offer independent childbirth education classes privately on a weekly basis to couples.

Following on from becoming a Childbirth educator Gaby trained in Hypnobirthing® and then as an Advanced Certified Hypnosis practitioner to assist her clients to release fear and anxiety and birth trauma, from a previous birth experience.

Due to necessity, need and desire by women wanting to become Doulas, Gaby wrote and implemented doula training, and in 2003 she ran the first official doula training course in Western Australia.

In 2004, Gabrielle attended the first Australian Doula conference in Sydney, followed by the 23rd Australian

Homebirth conference where she co-presented on the benefits of labouring and birthing in water from her perspective.

In 2005, Gaby launched her business, A Labour of Love, and released a pregnancy/labour range and Hypnosis for Birth Scripts available on iTunes.

A Labour of Love – Gabrielle Targett continues to be of services today providing online courses, webinars, and workshops to empower women and their partners all over the world.

Foreword

One of my research participants told me that she paid her doctor a heap of money to prop up the wall. She thought he was terrific because in no way did, he unnecessarily interfere with her birthing. The natural childbirth movement is about moving towards giving self-managed, safe and happy birthing totally back to women. It is also about giving men who know what they are doing an understanding of their vital role during natural birth, which is to see that women are free to have their babies happily and safely without any interference or any need to be concerned with what is happening in the world around them.

Gaby Targett, in her marvelously sensitive book, is moving western women back to the future in which pain will be rarely experienced and without need of any suppressive trance, let alone analgesia or anesthetics. The mechanism for painless delivery has already been biologically built in by mother nature in her basic design for birthing. Blood loss, if it happens, will be minimal. Tearing will be very rare even with relatively large babies and it will not matter much whether babies choose to arrive head or tail first. This is how it is for a number of 'primitive' peoples who, so far as birthing is concerned, are somewhat more civilised than we are.

In his book, *The Scientification of Love*, Michel Odent has said '... some topics of research have been regarded as politically incorrect by the medical establishment and have been deliberately neglected'. So, it is with Grantly Dick-Read's work. As his stepson, I find it very frustrating to see his writings so often misquoted and even distorted by people who will not search and accurately cite original documentation. In the introduction to the 2004 edition of Dick-Read's *Childbirth Without Fear*, Dr Odent has also said, 'Had lessons been learned from Grantly Dick-Read, the epidemic of malpractice suits and their consequences might have been prevented'. Gaby Targett's dream reflects my step- father's and it delights me so much to see how well she appreciates and honors his original contribution to the achievement of natural childbirth.

Leigh Dick-Read, 2005
MAppSc., Father, Natural Childbirth Educator,
Psychotherapist, PhD candidate researching natural childbirth

Contents

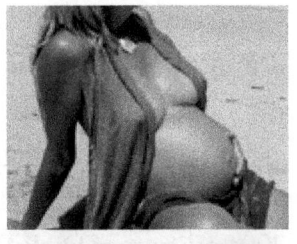
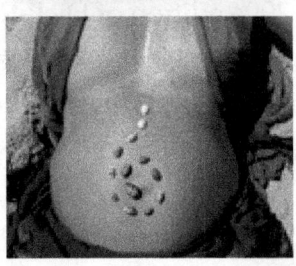

Preface	11
Introduction	13
1. In The Beginning – Where It All Began	17
2. A Little Inspiration	24
3. Positive Birth Preparation	43
4. You Have Many Options	50
5. It's Never Too Early Too Plan!	60
6. Having Sibling's Present	69
7. Preparing For Your Marathon Or Sprint	73
8. Optimal Foetal Position Makes A Labour Of Difference	94
9. The Power Of Pregnancy And Labour Hormones	109
10. Avoiding The Fear–Tension–Pain Syndrome	124

11. Understanding Your Uterus	129
12. Changing The Birthing Room To Suit Your Needs And Progress Your Labour	133
13. What Are The Benefits Of Having A Natural Childbirth?	138
14. Natural Pain-Relief Methods	143
15. Hypnosis For Birth Preparation	152
16. Opiate Pain Relief	157
17. Choosing And Educating Your Birth Support People	164
18. Doula Support	173
19. EDD – Estimated Due Date	180
20. What Do You Do When Labour Starts?	188
21. Established Labour	202
22. How To Prepare The Perineum	222
23. The Arrival Of Your Cherub	229
24. Breastfeeding	239
25. Pregnancy Topics Of Interest	255
26. Birth Stories	264
27. Estelle's Epilogue	321
Notes	326
References	329
Index	331

Preface

The nine months of pregnancy is a time of adjustment, and acceptance of the life force within; a time of education and acceptance of the changing body, mind and spirit; and a time to celebrate the journey into a new life and the *beautiful birth* ahead – none of which have a place for self-doubt or fear.

Empowered Birth and guide to childbirth without fear takes a non-medical approach. My knowledge and training come from attending many births throughout Western Australia. It is an open, honest account of information that women who are pregnant can use to create the type of birth experience they want. This book aims to empower women to believe in their bodies and themselves, so they may move forward through pregnancy feeling strong and excited about birth rather than anxious and fearful.

I want to assist women to look forward in a positive way and I want women to ask themselves, 'what type of birth do I want for my baby and my body'?

With the aim of empowering women around childbirth I aim to:

- Encourage women to look deep within.
- Cover the emotional aspects of childbirth.
- Look at the psychological aspects of birth;
- Describe the physical aspects of birth in a way that demystifies the fear of birth; and

- Question why there is so much fear around birth today.

Why this book is different to other books written about pregnancy and childbirth is because...

Empowered Birth covers exactly what you need to know to give birth, whether its your 1st or 3rd time around. Having knowledge and skills to physically and mentally prepare for labour are fundamental to create the birth you want and desire.

I highlight what is possible to achieve in any birthing situation: home, hospital or birthing centre. I have drawn from my own experience of three positive births, and from the experience of attending over 450 births over 28 years as a professional birth assistant.

I have seen every type of birth experience imaginable and have come to realise what really works for women and what does not.

At the end of the day what is important to remember is, you only get one opportunity to birth your baby into the world, and the choice is yours and yours alone as to how you decide to do it.

Love your way,
Gabrielle xx

Introduction

There are many reasons why I decided to write this book and finally get down on paper the thoughts, ideas and experiences I have been privileged to have gained during my own pregnancy, birthing and mothering journey. Not only have I acquired a wealth of information from my own experiences, but I have also gained insights from attending other women's births as a doula. For the first 10 years of witnessing birth as a doula my brain was exploding with information about birth. I have included material from nearly every birth I have attended, as for many years I have made notes based on my observations in order to truly understand birth.

First, let me say that I am not a writer by any means. I have written this book in 'lay' terms, as I am not medically trained. However, I am a person with knowledge and information to share about birth and I believe my perspective and my knowledge is important for pregnant women and their partners. I hope that you enjoy reading it as much as I have enjoyed labouring away over the years, the birth of my 'fourth baby' being the publishing of this book!

Let me begin by sharing with you my main reason for writing this book. When I wrote my first edition of this book in 2005, I wrote the reason I wanted to write this book was because of all the fear surrounding birth. Here I sit today, in 2021 renewing and rewriting the chapters and information and nothing has changed. The fear is even more prevalent and the induction rates off the chart, so more than ever women need the information and content in this book to help them trust and believe in their body that it can and will go into labour naturally but also to learn not to fear birth because it is one of the most empowering amazing experiences a women can go through. With the right empowered and positive education on board it can be ecstasy.

Women need to keep sharing birth stories that are positive and powerful to encourage others not so confident before natural birth becomes a thing of the past and no longer be an option. Intervention and the medical approach to birthing have become the 'norm'. Women are rapidly losing their ability and power to have the wonderful birth experience they deserve. So often today, women hand all their care and all responsibility of birthing over to someone else, without giving any consideration to their rights, choice or belief in their body.

It terrifies me to think my daughter, Jaeosha, may never have the opportunity to experience childbirth naturally, in her place of choice, without having to go into hospital if she so wishes. *Childbirth is about choice.* I believe a woman should be given the choice and right to say what she believes and have her choices honored by all who surround her on her baby's birthday. This is known as the 'BIRTHRIGHT' of the mother and the baby: for the child to be brought into the world in a gentle and natural way. I distinctly remember after the birth of my second son, Jarrad, Jaeosha turned to me and said, 'Mum, I want to have a baby come out of my wooza [the name we used for vagina] in the water just like you, when I have a baby.' She was four years old at the time. From time to time we still talk at great length about birth, and what it looks like and how it feels. To this day Jaeosha mentions to me how she would like to birth her babies, when her time comes around. She is 27 now and so many of her friends are having babies led by the techno-medical model of birth resulting in high intervention. This seems to be the norm now for many women, but it still does not have to be this way. Just know with the right education, belief and empowerment you will always have a choice, unless that one variable arises that you didn't foresee coming and you are required and willing to go down the medical route for the safety of you and bubs.

As birthing currently stands in Australia and other countries around the globe, there is a lack of resolution of insurance issues, which is eliminating independently working midwives from practice, as they are not able to find a company willing to insure them. This is a particularly difficult situation for private home- birth midwives, who are truly experts in the field of birthing. Other major issues surrounding birth include doctors not wanting to take risks, high-risk women being offered Caesarean sections, the impending loss of government-sponsored homebirth midwifery programs, and obstetric care in the hospital being seen as the norm.

These are issues of real concern. The current trends will affect our daughters and their daughters, and their daughters that follow. I very much feel that women need to collectively work together, to take ownership and responsibility, and to take charge of birth once again, to change the current trends in child- birth and the beliefs women have about birth. What will women have in the future as a choice if we as a collective don't do something now to improve the concept of childbirth? If we don't act immediately, there may come a time when women just don't birth naturally. That is something I cannot bear to think about. Where would the world be without natural birth being available as a realistic option?

To articulate my dream, let me use the words of Dr Grantly Dick-Read. Back in 1942 he wrote:

> *The imagery of childbirth will no longer be clouded by mystery and anguish. The adolescent girl will not whisper disturbing hearsay to her friends, but seek to value, fashion and protect her mind and body so that she may, in fullness of time, be fitted and untarnished to take her place with serenity and pride amongst the chosen women of her time.*

1

In The Beginning – Where It All Began

My passion about childbirth came from some inspiring people whom I was very fortunate to meet at the tender age of twenty-three, when I lived in Tokyo for one year, a year that changed my life. I am a great believer in being in the right place at the right time, and Japan was no exception. To this day, I believe my whole purpose in being in Tokyo was not to work as a swimming instructor, but to meet a vast array of amazing people that got me onto my path and life journey. A journey working with women, to assist them to birth and teach them the way forward into the unfamiliar world of natural childbirth.

When I think back, it was really no coincidence that my life and destiny changed while living in Japan. The experience opened so many doors and gave me new learning opportunities, which led me to discovering my passions in life: water birth, natural birth, swimming with dolphins and babyswim – all of which I knew nothing about when I arrived in Japan.

My first experience started with a friend calling me up one day and saying in her American accent, 'Hey Gaby, would you like to come and hear this obstetrician guy called Michel Odent at a conference next week?'

'Yeah, sounds fantastic,' I replied.

'He is going to talk about water birth and his work in the UK and Europe.'

'I am there,' I said.

And so my journey began, even though I didn't really know it at that time.

I went to Michel Odent's conference, excited but not really knowing what to expect. As I entered one of Tokyo's tall buildings I moved into the elevator, where I turned to meet the eyes of Michel Odent in the lift. Initially I didn't have a clue who he was, but through our exchange of words it soon became evident. From that moment I sensed that I was in the right place at the right time, that somewhere in the scheme of things I needed to be in that lift talking to Michel, connecting with one of the world's leading obstetric professionals. Right from the outset I felt his strong passion and commitment to his work and research and was sure this conference was going to be very insightful and life-changing in many ways.

During Michel's conference he showed many water-birth footage to Japanese obstetricians, midwives and general practitioners, all of whom were very impressed. On that day, for the very first time, I too saw a water birth, and I knew in my heart that if and when I fell pregnant, I would be bringing my baby into the world in the water. And in 1995, 1997 and 1999 I did just that! I had three water births, each two years and one month apart, almost to the day. I strongly believe the reason I was able to have such powerful and positive water-birth experiences was due to that chance meeting and attendance at the conference with Michel Odent. This is where I was really shown what birth could look like and made to feel empowered – that I could birth naturally in the water if I wanted to. It felt as though Michel's passion and understanding of birth rubbed off onto me and got under my skin.

My next learning experience and life-changing event occurred upon meeting another amazing person during my time in Japan. Estelle Myers came to the swimming club where I worked and ran a series of fun, uplifting, relaxing aquatic workshops – including baby swim training – for the staff. Estelle is an amazing spokesperson and advocate for releasing dolphins and whales who are kept in captivity. She was in the process of trying to free Corky the killer whale in San Diego when I met her, and her other achievements include setting up the first ever human/dolphin research centre in New Zealand. Estelle was inspired to investigate the possibility of birthing human babies from the waters of the womb into the waters of the world, like our ocean-going cousins the dolphins.

In 1982 in New Zealand, Estelle began supporting water births, which were the first in the southern hemisphere at that time. The women who were water birthing their babies with Estelle and the midwives were considered to be quite radical back then, being that there were at that time only about 100 water births in the world.

In 1985 Estelle went to Russia and met with Igor Charkovsky, renowned for his work with water births and babies swimming from birth in the home bath. Then, in the freezing waters of Gorky Park, Estelle witnessed toddlers and children swimming in the middle of winter, with snow all around. Estelle's primary aim in going to Russia was to find out exactly what this extraordinary man was doing in Moscow. As a result of her visit and filming she went on to promote his teachings and beliefs through making a documentary of his work, in an attempt to let the world know of the possibilities of the human baby.

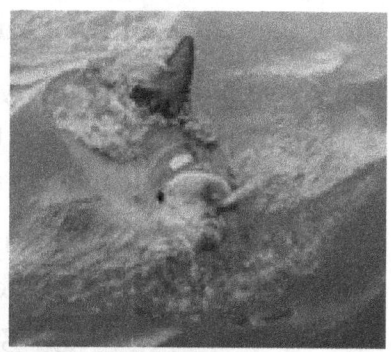

After eight years of commitment towards promoting water birth and baby-swimming around the globe, in 1990 Estelle won the United Nations Media Peace Prize for the documentary *Oceania: The Promise of Tomorrow*. This film integrated all that she had seen, all the amazing people she had met and, most importantly, informed people about baby-swimming and waterbirth (as well as addressing the needs of understanding how dolphins and whales live in the wild and in captivity). The essence Estelle emits from her personality, in real life and on film, is that life is about fun and play and cooperation, and that love of life is an essential ingredient for happiness.

My overall impression of this gung-ho person was that she could make the impossible seem possible. And after our encounter together in Japan we forged a strong and dynamic friendship, which to this day still exists. I feel so fortunate that my eyes were opened and before me was a woman imparting all of her knowledge, beliefs and understandings on subject areas that beautifully intertwined with my own interests and beliefs, which led on to this amazing birth journey of my own.

Not only did Estelle impart her knowledge and beliefs about baby-swimming to me, but I also had the opportunity of experiencing my first swim with wild dolphins when Estelle introduced me to members of a Japanese-based dolphin interaction group who took me to an island off the coast of Japan for my first close encounter! This was an amazing and uplifting experience and one that I have pursued regularly for the past twelve years, especially during my pregnancies. It is true that dolphins are very attracted to pregnant women and can always sense when they are around.

Swimming with wild dolphins requires total trust and acceptance of yourself with the dolphins and the dolphins with you. Through your body language and actions, which need to be free and uninhibited, one gains a sense of trust, elation and freedom, where fear has no part to play when swimming with these wild, wonderful creatures. What makes this experience so incredibly special and unique is, firstly, both you and the dolphin are on equal terms in the watery environment – freely suspended in neutral territory. Secondly, there is a degree of curiosity between each other. When a dolphin in the wild chooses to swim over and make eye contact in a totally trusting way, it is amazing to say the least. The senses are overcome with feelings of love, peace, happiness and playfulness, not to mention trust. These are very similar feelings to those of labour and childbirth.

Like the dolphins' love of their aquatic environment, Estelle too displayed a love of life, peace, happiness and playfulness. Estelle's *Oceania* film shows the peace that babies experience when they have come into the world via waterbirth. When babies are born from the waters of the womb into the waters of the world, the transition from one to another results in calm and peaceful human beings. Could this possibly be the solution to world peace?

When I had first arrived in Japan, I'd felt like an empty vessel; when I left Japan to head back to Australia the empty vessel was full to the brim! I had renewed energy and excitement and was bursting to get back and live my life according to my new philosophy. Firstly, though, I wanted to find some dolphin friends to swim with, and secondly, find a new man to have a baby with, and thirdly – of course – to experience a water birth.

Like most things in my life, everything fell into place easily. Back in Australia, I returned to university to finish my Physical Education degree. Two months after returning I met my husband-to-be, Jerome. We spent the next couple of years getting to know one another and went on to have three children, all born in the water with a private midwife. I want to share my stories for the simple reason that I want others to know that my experience of childbirth was wonderful. It is important for women to share positive birthing experiences, so other women feel empowered, and therefore ready to create their own birth desires and wishes. Although I had three water births, each was very different from the other and special in its own unique way.

I believe that 'our thoughts really do create our reality', so if you put a clear enough request forward you can create anything. This is how I approached the birth of my first baby. I didn't read many books or listen to any negative stories, only positive ones. I remember just asking lots of questions of my doctor and my amazingly gifted midwife, Mary Murphy.

With each and every birth I knew I was bringing into the world another human being, different from any other on the planet. That is a very profound concept.

Thanks to Michel Odent, who had etched into my memory the waterbirth scenes from his videos, I visualised on a daily basis what my birth was going to look like. I also attended a very informative yoga class where I learned what I needed to know through open discussion with other women. Some might call this type of preparation a little light, or downright stupid, but I just knew I didn't want to listen to any negative and irrelevant information, of which there was so much around at that time.

So, by the time I came to birth my first baby I felt strong, both physically and mentally, as I had given a lot of thought and consideration to mental preparation, and physically I was fit and healthy from participating in yoga and teaching aqua-aerobics throughout my entire pregnancy. I had all my questions answered and I was empowered by those around me to believe and trust in my body to do the very job it is designed to do, with not a doubt in my mind. This, I felt, was the key to creating a positive natural birth experience, which happened to be in the water.

2
A Little Inspiration

The day before the estimated due date of my first baby I desperately wanted to drive down to Bunbury, three hours south of Perth, Western Australia, to have a swim with my friends the dolphins. Since returning from Japan I was a regular swimmer in the waters of Bunbury with my flippered pals, thanks to my good friend Rowena, whom I met in Bunbury. Rowena became my constant swimming companion with the dolphins. Over the years since my return from Japan, we had experienced some awesome and unforgettable interactions that we hold in our memories and hearts forever. Some dolphins I befriended, particularly females in the pods, who would always come and show me their babies. When I was pregnant I had a strong sense that they knew I was carrying a baby, as their interaction times increased and they seemed to intensify their visits with me whenever I entered the water.

On that day in April 1995, I got into the water and had the most amazing interaction with the dolphins. They were all around myself and Jerome. I frolicked and dived and did somersaults for hours with them. At times, I just floated and they cruised slowly under me while I relaxed and caught my breath; being heavily pregnant the dolphins' pace and excitement tired me out quickly.

I was at peace and content and reassured by their presence. At one stage they jumped out of the water over Jerome and I as if to express their pure delight and excitement for the interaction and experience. I really think the dolphins sensed that I was very close to birthing the baby I was carrying.

I arrived home from our outing to Bunbury feeling uplifted, energised and physically tired. I rang my midwife, Mary, to tell her that I was back in one piece from our amazing adventure and that I was so glad to have gone down to the dolphins, because now I felt ready to birth. On that note she suggested I go to bed early to get some sleep.

At 4 a.m. in the morning I was woken by a trickle of water coming out of my body. I sat up, saying to Jerome, 'I think my waters have just broken.' I stood up and with that the biggest gush of water left my body. 'Yep, it's my waters all right,' and with that I walked to the bathroom to get a towel to clean up the liquid on the floor. I went back to bed unfazed about my waters breaking and tried to get some sleep. I found sleeping impossible, as I knew I was going to be having a baby that day and I was so excited.

I rang Mary about 7 a.m. to tell her my waters had broken. She explained that she couldn't get to me till 1 p.m. so she would send around a backup midwife, Bronwyn Key, to check on me. At 11 a.m. Bronwyn came over to check my progress and to have a cup of tea. All was well, and I just plodded around the house with the period cramping I was feeling, which was getting stronger and stronger by the hour. I had at the back of my mind that I had to wait for Mary to arrive before I could go into proper labour – whatever proper labour was! I guess to some degree I was holding back from actually allowing myself to really get into the swing of strong contractions as I wanted Mary to be there. I was not complaining, however, as I had a lovely warm-up which helped prepare me physically and mentally for the labour that was to follow.

On the dot, Mary arrived with her big hug and reassuring smile. It was a relief to see her, because at long last I could let go and allow myself to go into proper labour, and I did. Like clockwork the contractions started to intensify and hold me up from walking freely around the room. At 2.30 p.m. Mary suggested I get into our normal oval-shaped bath for a little natural pain relief. For all of ten minutes I stayed in the bath, as I found that sitting on my bottom with my legs out straight was agony. I could not cope at all with the contractions and I told Mary so in no uncertain terms.

Women in labour need not worry about what they say to others in labour, and need to be forgiven for the way in which they speak, and for what they may say out of heightened intensity. This is the right of a labouring woman.

I moved from the bathroom to the papasan chair in the bedroom. At last I felt comfortable! At about 4 p.m. I remember saying, 'Mary, I really need to do a poo!' She replied in her very casual manner, 'That's OK, I have my poo-catcher here, I will just catch it.' I was thinking, 'Wow! What a woman to catch my poo!' But at that point Mary called for Jerome. I noticed a little quiver in her voice which suggested this was urgent – she told Jerome to quickly go to Woodside Hospital and set up the proper birthing tub as I was going to need it very soon.

I was heading to Woodside, our local maternity hospital, as I have a blood disorder called Von Willebrand's Disease, which means my blood has problems clotting. In my case, the specialists weren't sure if I was going to bleed abnormally and have a haemorrhage. Just in case, we had planned to go to the hospital towards the end of my labour, to experience my water birth, where they had clotting factors waiting for me in case I needed it. (As it turned out I didn't, and all was fine.)

So I watched Jerome take off in the car to go and set up the tub. I realised that my friend (another Gabrielle!), who was to be my birth support person, was still down the street in my car with the screws and bolts to put the birth tub together! There was nothing I could do but pray that somehow she would be back in time for the birth. In the meantime, I was getting louder and louder in my noises and Mary suggested we also get to the hospital in her car.

I can tell you that it was easier said than done! Heading down the stairs I was trying to put on a dress and have a contraction at the same time! I can remember that the journey down those stairs seemed to take forever. When I finally arrived at the bottom step I burst out of the house and onto the front lawn for all the neighbours to see, my ass in the air, and me yelling, 'Mary, just leave me here, I want to have the baby here!' With that she picked me up and got me into the car for the quickest drive around the neighbourhood I had ever experienced. Suddenly, like a miracle, we arrived at Woodside's back door.

I learnt an important lesson during this birth, which was just how essential it is that you are clear with your support people, explaining to them prior to the birth exactly what it is you expect from them and what is appropriate and not appropriate at any time.

I again flung myself out of the car and onto the lawn. I presume this is a regular occurrence for the locals who live across the road from this maternity hospital – a woman in labour, on all fours, yelling something obscene to the driver of the car!

Yet again Mary lifted me up and told me that under no circumstances was a baby going to be born on the lawn outside the hospital. She marched me inside telling me to pant. Inside I saw Jerome and Gabrielle madly trying to get the tub ready while I laboured on the bed. Gabrielle wanted to show me the dolphin photos from the day before, thinking I would find this calming and relaxing. At this point I have to say all I wanted was to get into the tub and push.

Looking at dolphin photos lasted about thirty seconds and then the need to push became so overwhelming that all I could think about was the tub, water and the birth.

At about 4.20 p.m. I got into the tub, which was wonderful. At that moment I felt calm, relaxed and again able to surrender to what was happening to my body. I had about four contractions where I pushed really hard and my baby pushed out to her ears. At this point all I could feel was the 'Chinese Burn' sensation in my perineum as it stretched. Mary supported the baby's head, which allowed my perineum to expand and give. I then had another really intense contraction where I made the most amazing noise like a primal animal. It bellowed out of me from deep within and seemed to echo through the room and down the corridor. With that sound, I pushed Jaeosha out of my body in one push, and she slipped through the water over to the other side of the tub as if swimming.

Our journey together was just beginning, and I felt we had got off to a great start with the most amazingly fast, positive and beautiful birth experience, that I just loved!

It was 4.32 p.m. when Jaeosha rocketed out of my body. Mary had to move over to the other side of the tub to pick her up and she placed her gently on my chest. I remember saying, 'Look, it is a baby. I can't believe I have had a baby.' I am not sure what I thought the outcome would be!

With Jaeosha on my chest we sat for what seemed like an eternity, just looking at each other, looking deep into each other's eyes. The weight of her body, the warmth, smell and softness of her skin were beautiful and uplifting. At last we had met face to face, skin to skin.

I got out of the tub to deliver the placenta, which I have to say felt like a big wet jellyfish sliding out! Having had Jaeosha so quickly I had little trouble in expelling the placenta. The only downside to a really fast birth is occasionally the body goes into shock, and this is what happened with me. I had a really high temperature and was sweating profusely, and my blood pressure was high, all symptoms which are not unusual after a quick birth. Something I hadn't counted on was having very strong after-birth contractions, which really blew me away. Every time I went to breastfeed Jaeosha the contractions became so intense that I had to breathe slowly just to get through them, just like I had done during the labour. For a while I really thought that maybe, just maybe, I was having twins and I had forgotten about the other one! These afterbirth pains went on for about three days, all of which is considered normal with very quick births, but is more likely to occur with second and third births than the first.

Although my first experience was fast, I have to say it was indeed a positive birth and one I will always remember clearly. The first time any woman births, the experience is so new that every sensation is observed and analysed with your conscious mind. And often lots of questioning goes on internally. Is this supposed to happen? Is that OK? And so on. These thoughts and feelings are all very normal and to a certain degree teach and prepare us for the next experience. If there is a next experience. In my case I knew there was going to be.

During their second labour experience women often relax a little more, knowing they have a fair idea of just what to expect and that there is light at the end of the tunnel. After all the hard work the birth of a baby is the end result. Sometimes women actually forget that this is the true purpose of labour, as I seemed to during Jaeosha's birth. Despite this fact, having had a positive first experience does prepare women to look forward to the next with great anticipation, as I did.

My Second Birth Journey

The second of my births started like my first with the 4 a.m. wake-up call. However, this time it was a very strong contraction that woke me. I waddled to the toilet in readiness for my waters breaking, but to my dismay this didn't happen. I had looked forward to this unusual sensation and wanted this to be the real thing as I was ten days over my supposed due date and getting very heavy and tired. I went back to bed having mild period-pain-type contractions that kept me in a half-sleep and half-conscious state, my brain mulling over the fact that today I was going to have a baby.

The excitement once again set in and I found it hard to get any more rest.

At about 7 a.m. I rang Mary, the same midwife I had had for Jaeosha's birth, to tell her of my contractions. Mary had in the back of her mind that I would be having a pretty fast labour, and said she would be straight over, as soon as she showered. I then took to walking the streets block by block to get things moving along. Walking the streets in early labour always reminds me of a friend who lived in Alice Springs who walked through the labours of her four children and as a consequence had very quick, easy births. This inspired me to do the same and off I headed. I always wondered what people thought of a big, heavy pregnant woman walking the streets with a towel slung over her shoulder.

What you may ask is the towel for? Just in case the waters break! Stopping to have contractions, leaning on people's fences can be very entertaining, especially if noises are coming from your throat deep within, as you puff and pant through a contraction. This can draw people out to come and see what is going on. Just smile and carry on your way!

I walked and walked till I felt it was time to move my labouring body back to the house for Mary to check my baby's foetal heart rate and have a feel of the baby's head from the outside, to see how far down it was into the pelvis. All was going well, and I wandered around the house going to the toilet as often as I could to relieve my bladder, which was being squashed flat like a pancake by the baby's head pushing down.

In my anxiousness to go into labour I had set up the timber frame of the birthing tub the day before, in readiness for the birth and to try to spur it on both physically and subconsciously. (We were having this baby at home.) As I wandered about the house having the odd strong contraction, I started to get anxious about getting the soft foam and liners into the tub's frame, ready for the water. Oh the water! How I dreamed, leading up to this birth, about wallowing around and really enjoying the sensation of the water for a much longer time. In hindsight we really do have to watch what we ask for, as I got just that, a much longer time!

After many trips to the toilet to check on the show (mucus plug or bloody show as it is often referred to) in my undies, many games of UNO – a great card game – and a really funny laughing session looking at Gary Larson's *Far Side* calendar, I finally went into proper labour. Proper labour is known as established labour, and you really have to concentrate on each and every contraction, usually by closing your eyes and burying your face. After a substantial period of time in established labour, Mary felt I was far enough along to get into the birthing tub. By hopping into the tub too early, I could have slowed down or even stopped the contractions. This is always a possibility as water is so relaxing that the body sometimes responds by relaxing a little too much.

Once immersed in the water I felt the intensity of the contractions being reduced so I could work with my body and surrender completely, and not fight natural rhythmical waves opening my body and flowing through me.

I stripped off as fast as I could and dived in. Well, I would have dived in had my belly allowed me that privilege! Once in the water I felt at peace with my body and relieved to have the weight off my feet, legs, pubic bone and pelvis. At last I could float totally suspended if I wanted to. The best part about being in the water was that when the contractions really started to get tough I could surrender and work with my body, not against it.

Once in the tub, that is where I stayed, from 2 p.m. in the afternoon until my baby arrived into the world a little over four hours later. Apart from wanting a longer birth and more time in the tub (and I certainly got that!), this time I distinctly remember going through the transition stages of labour.

It has been noted in many books that transition is a time when a labouring woman gets really shitty, swears and feels very hot and sometimes abusive to anyone around her for a short duration of time acting totally out of character. This is due to the adrenaline sweeping through her body!

For me, transition was marked by sharply telling SusanJane, Mary's apprentice home-birth midwife at the time, to stop massaging me. I remember snarling, 'Don't touch me, just leave me alone.' With that I went and sat myself in the middle of the tub where no one could reach me. I then said to Mary, 'I just want this baby out of me now, get it out, I have had enough.'

Mary looked at SusanJane in a knowing sort of way and both said 'transition' in unison.

Afterwards I apologised, as I felt incredibly rude–SusanJane had been massaging me for about four hours continuously before I reached transition and I had found it incredibly calming, not to mention wonderful having pressure on my lower back and pelvis. Just after the end of my transitional stage it was as if a miracle had happened. The intensity 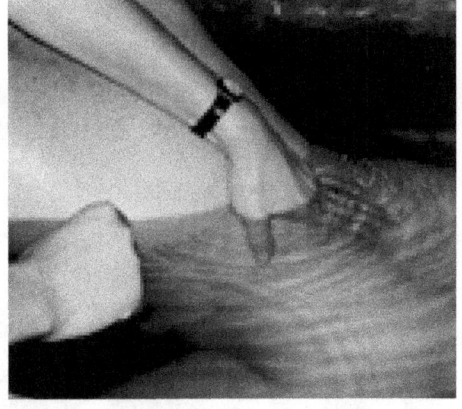 had shifted in my body from deep within my pelvis, cervix and vagina to my bottom, where once again I felt the need to do a poo. Oh, the poo sensation, how I longed to feel this again. It was a welcome sensation, as I knew at this point, with the urge to push, I was nearly at the end of my marathon and had about two kilometres to go to get to the finish line. The only problem was I was hitting the wall fast. I knew I just had to keep going, so on I worked, and pushed, and vocalised rather loudly. The raw energy and adrenalin of birth once again supported me and saw me through. At last I was having a moment of 'runner's high', and it was great!

The pushing sensation took over my whole body and, as in my first labour, not pushing was impossible once the urge came on. I felt this was a big baby and Mary was coaching me, sensitive to the fact that I was getting pretty close to pushing this baby out. We had previously discussed that when the time came and the head was pushing through my perineum I would take it easy and pant and resist pushing, and really listen to what Mary was saying, if I could. This would prevent my perineum from tearing badly. Mindful of tearing I made the effort to pant like an animal in the wild giving birth! Then, without any consideration or thought on my behalf, my waters broke. This sounded like the cork on a champagne bottle flying off, for all in the room to hear. The celebration of birth had begun and I was overjoyed that soon I could be drinking real champagne to celebrate.

At last the 'Chinese Burn' came and lasted for what seemed like an eternity, but, as requested by Mary, I panted through the next contraction so the perineum could retract and slide back over the baby on its own. With the next contraction, as with Jaeosha's birth, I expected my baby's body to fly out of me. Well, not with this baby! I had to work him out on every contraction, to the point where he was hanging out of my body, totally stuck with my perineum around his stomach, as he was so large around his midriff. I ended up saying, 'Mary, can you please just pull the baby out, I've had enough.' With that he slipped out calmly and peacefully into the water at 6.16 p.m. on the 16th day of May in 1997.

I attempted to turn around, so I could hold my baby, but I kept getting caught up in his very long umbilical cord. I actually had to lift my leg high into the air to get up and over it, so I could at last sit down and cuddle him. We were finally able to meet face to face and skin to skin. Words cannot even describe this moment. All I can say is that when you look into your baby's eyes for the first time it is the most wonderful moment a mother can experience, making the bond and connection very strong on every level possible.

I looked with Jerome and Jaeosha who had both been amazing birth support to see what sex this baby was. He had boy written all over him. By gee he was a boy. He had huge testicles and a penis that would make any man proud! The large size, due to swelling and hormones, is quite normal, Mary told me after his birth. The reason the boys look so well-endowed is because of the amount of blood that flows to the genitals during the birth. Boys' genitals do go down after the birth, to be more in proportion with the rest of their body.

Benjamin, as we named him, was a good eight and a half pounds of muscle; he was solid but chubby. Best of all he was so healthy and happy-looking that I just wanted to eat him all up. Your own baby always looks so scrumptious and has the most incredible baby smell. Yummy.

Finally, I got out of the tub to deliver the placenta, as I had done before, and to be monitored for blood loss. Right on cue the placenta slipped out like a big jellyfish, all soft and squishy! It was a delight to have finished the process of giving birth and have Jerome finally cut the cord. This, to me, symbolised all the work I had done and the journey I was to start, as mother, provider of food, protector and nurturer for the years to come. To me, the birth represents the beginning of the process of life together as mother and child. 'Wow, a boy. My baby boy, Ben.'

My Third Birth Journey

Once again the sharp pains of contractions at 4 a.m. in the morning disturbed my sleep. I don't know what it is about 4 a.m. in the morning and going into labour, but that is how and when my labours all started. I got up on this very cold morning in June and decided to light the fire, so I set about chopping wood and getting the kindling alight in the open fireplace. I imagined that this is how it must have been for women in early Australian settlers' times: lighting the fire and doing the odd job, knowing that a baby was going to be born on that day.

I did some exercises and yoga in front of the fire to try to get things going. I was eight days 'overdue' and really BIG. This time I wanted a birth that was not as long as Benjamin's, as that felt like it had been a little too long! In my head I was requesting a three-hour birth. This I knew I could do. After some time in front of the fire I decided to go back to bed as I again felt tired and thought maybe I should get some rest before the big event.

At 6 a.m. the contractions were starting to feel really intense when I was lying down, so I got out of bed. The intensity surprised me as I thought that I would have more of the period type of pain as a warm-up before I got to this point. I decided at this stage that I had better phone Mary. Once again, Mary Murphy was supporting me with her excellent midwifery skills. I think she felt this was going to be a fast labour, as she said, 'I'll jump in the shower and be right over in twenty minutes!' This amused me as she lived about thirty-five to forty minutes away. I had visions of a speeding midwife on the freeway zooming through all the cars that slowed her down, waving her hand and yelling, 'Get out of my way.' All in the name of birth!

This birth was another planned homebirth, with both Jaeosha (now four) and Ben (now two) with us at home. In the time it took Mary to arrive, I proceeded to start to labour. My only problem was that Benjamin was driving me crazy. With each contraction he saw, he wanted to be picked up and cuddled by me. Some two- year-olds do not understand what is happening when they see Mummy in labour and can get needy. This was happening to Ben. As soon as I could muster up the energy I blurted out to Jerome, 'Phone the neighbours to come and get Ben, right now please.'

When I finally saw Ben walk down the driveway holding my neighbour's hand, I could stop trying to hold myself together.

Pam England and Rob Horowitz refer to this in their book *Birthing from Within* as 'performance anxiety'. They suggest that external factors, such as being watched while in labour, can slow a woman down, due to the subconscious mind telling your body that you are not feeling very comfortable about your situation. This is exactly how I felt with Ben being in close proximity to me. I knew the only way to stop this was to get him out of the house.

Another lesson I learned about women is they should never have to hold back and not do what their body wants to do. As this is not surrendering to the natural process of labour and will ultimately interfere with dilation progress.

I walked back into the house and headed for the bathroom to take up my favourite position of burying my face into the towels on the towel rack while groaning and grunting. I asked to get into the tub, however the tub wasn't quite ready. Also, a needle in the bum had to happen first. I was dreading this more than anything, and in fact felt I could handle contractions any day over 100 millilitres of antibiotic in the backside while in labour!

I will digress here to explain the reason I had to have the antibiotic. I had a condition called Strep B. No one is sure how I picked it up and it is only really dangerous when you have large quantities of the bacteria in your vagina around birth time. I'd had it three times previously throughout this pregnancy, so it was not a shock when on my due date, after having yet another internal swab, I knew I had it again.

With Strep B, there is a risk that the baby could be born with the Strep B bacteria, as it can pass from the mother's fluids into the baby's mouth, nose or eyes and they can become very sick. At the time of this birth, the protocol to manage Strep B included: immediately after birth the contents of the baby's stomach to be sucked out and sent off to the lab and tested, and strong antibiotics to be given to both the mother and baby by injection. This can be enough to stop the baby from getting very sick, and in my case it was, thank goodness!

Boy, did I squeal like a pig when the dreaded injection went in. I think it was because I was so close to transition and my entire body of nerve endings was on alert due to the intensity of the contractions. I have to say I also hate needles! With the jab over and done with, I bolted from the bed and into the tub. That was the pay-off for having the injection and being brave. Once again I slid into the tub and felt at home. A sensation of peace and tranquillity swept over my body as my great friend Sue put her warm and loving hands onto my back and started massaging. Sue massaged me till the end of my labour, and for this I am eternally grateful.

The labour intensified even more when I got into the tub. The edge was taken off the top of each contraction due to being immersed in the water and having massage; however, they were still pretty intense and occurring very rapidly with lots of piggy- back contractions. These are contractions that are very strong and come one after the other consecutively, with no rest in between. It was at this stage I remember saying 'Fuuuuuuuuck', drawing out the sound as long and hard as I could. What I was trying to do was find a sound I could identify with and use to help me get this baby out. All that kept going through my brain was Fuuuuuuuuck.

Jerome suggested that I try another word, as he was concerned that with Jaeosha present at the birth, she might start to imitate that sound and word after the birth. However, Mary suggested that it didn't even sound like the actual word and to keep going as it was helping me to open up incredibly. I remember at one stage looking over at Jaeosha as she whispered in my ear, 'It's OK, Mummy, you are going to have the baby soon.' With that she placed a cold towel on my forehead and kissed me. It was one of the most moving parts of the whole labour. Incredible to think that a four-year-old could acknowledge what was going on and totally support me in every conceivable way. This I will always remember.

Before long I was pushing and working really hard. This puzzled me, as my contractions were five minutes apart. I remember asking, 'Mary, how can I be pushing? My contractions are still five minutes apart.' As always, Mary reassured me that it was totally possible, and my body needed the time in between contractions to rest and recuperate, before the next one came.

With this change in stages it was time to call my attending doctor, who was needed to oversee the actual birth and the procedure that the baby had to undergo for the Strep B. The urge to push became stronger and stronger and before I knew it my baby's head was pushing on my perineum. Just as with Ben's birth my waters broke again, sending a loud popping sound out into the room for all to hear. My children loved coming into this world with a pop!

Mary supported me once again by reminding me to pant as my perineum stretched as I worked at taking it easy, so as not to push too quickly or forcefully. Having a midwife coach you through this stage can really help avoid a big tear and keep the perineum in great condition. My eyes remained totally closed for this part of the birth as I felt I just had to focus all my thoughts and feelings inwardly and really concentrate on the business at hand. I did squeeze Jerome's hand so hard that his rings actually cut into his skin, which I figure is a small price for a father to pay during childbirth!

Within five minutes and with two really strong pushes I had birthed my baby into the water at 9.30 a.m. Once again, I turned slowly around to feel his warm soft skin as he was placed on my body, which assisted with melting away the memory of the intensity of contractions that I had experienced only minutes before. All was forgotten in an instant, and all I could do was look at this incredibly beautiful angel-like figure on my chest. I was in love.

Together we sat in the tub just looking at each other. Jaeosha kissed and kissed his tiny little head. Someone suggested that Jerome and I look at the genitals to see what the sex of the baby was, so we did. At first I said, 'Oh, it's a girl', then someone suggested that I look again. To my surprise, (I thought I was having a girl) this baby was actually a boy! He looked so small and perfect with amazingly beautiful eyes that seemed to follow me everywhere. I felt totally connected with him on a very deep level.

I turned and asked Jerome if I could have some lunch, as I was starving. 'Lunch? Don't you mean breakfast?' said Mary. 'It is only 9.30 a.m. in the morning.' I was really surprised with this reply as I thought that I had laboured for a lot longer than in reality I had. I was totally oblivious to any sense of time, and had no clocks or watches around me. I have always done this with my births, because I believe time has no relevance where birth is concerned. It was finally time to hop out of the tub and onto the floor, where I then delivered the placenta. The cord was clamped and cut by Jerome when it had stopped pulsating. Jarrad, as we named him, was bundled up in towels, beanie and booties, ready for the tube down his throat and suction of his stomach. The downside to this was I didn't get to breastfeed him immediately, as I had done with Jaeosha and Ben. This first suckle can really help with the bonding that a mother and newborn share immediately after birth, as well as beginning to establish breastfeeding. To me, this first feed is always a special memory and moment. But, in this case, I had to put it on hold temporarily.

I couldn't watch the procedure take place. I was in the room, however. The thought of not being able to see him or hear him made me aware of just how painful it must be for parents to have their newborn baby taken away for tests or to another room immediately after birth. The feeling of loss must be incredible.

Jarrad was finally passed back to me, where Mary had set me up with lots of pillows, nice and snuggly on the couch in front of the fire. It was here he had his first feed and I dressed him in his new suit, which was pink! I had honestly thought I was having a girl and was a little shocked when I had looked again, to see that he was in fact a boy!

I thought to myself, if only all women could experience how great they can feel after a natural birth, the fear aspect would be completely gone forever. I was high from the birth and high on life, and overjoyed and content that my last birth experience could finish on such a positive and empowering note!

After the birth I felt fantastic. This was due to the cocktail of natural opiates my body was producing during the final stages of labour. After a couple of hours' rest I decided to take a shower, in which I felt even better than I had with Jae's and Ben's births. I didn't even feel sore through my perineum and there was absolutely no stinging from a graze or anything. I ended up walking around for a little bit doing the odd job around the house, in disbelief that I had just given birth to an eight-and-a-half-pound baby.

3
Positive Birth Preparation

My Preparation Story

In hindsight, I can see that I totally immersed myself in the positive aspects of birth. I actually went into the first birth having read only two books. One was, you guessed it, *Water Birth*, written by Janet Balaskas and Yehudi Gordon. The other book was one that tells you basically what you should be experiencing for how many weeks pregnant you are, written by Clark Gillespie. I really didn't read any further than that.

However, I did attend a wonderful yoga class at a place known as the Family Nurturing Centre, right on the beach with ocean views in Swanbourne, on the coast of Western Australia. I distinctly remember turning up to the class every week in my dreamy hormonal state, looking out across the ocean and seeing beautiful dolphins playing in the water, wishing I too could be out there playing with them. Through my first pregnancy I felt a strong connection with the dolphins, with water, and most importantly with myself – physically, mentally, emotionally and spiritually.

A labour of love

Sam and Sydel Weinstein run the Family Nurturing Centre yoga classes that I attended during my first pregnancy. Here I obtained a lot of my positive and valuable educational informtion and beliefs about childbirth – from a man, no less! Sam has his heart in the right place and is committed to helping women really trust their body and not get caught up with all of today's politics surrounding birth. It was through the weekly yoga sessions, and especially sitting around on the yoga mats after each class, that I was able to hear women talk about their births and how life was as a parent of a new baby.

I believed 100% my body could do the job it was designed to do without a doubt.

I feel privileged to have been exposed to an atmosphere that promoted open and honest stories first-hand, as well as support and encouragement for those who had not yet birthed. This was also the place where I first witnessed women openly breastfeeding and assisting other women who were having difficulties breastfeeding or other problems to do with being a mum for the first time. It was truly a place that nurtured women, who then nurtured and assisted others, something that our society needs more of!

The yoga helped my body to become strong, and the talking and listening helped me mentally prepare. I feel this is the best type of education women can experience for learning what is ahead of them. Being in a supported, nurturing environment where women can openly express themselves is so incredibly empowering in preparing women for the journey ahead into motherhood. Fathers too were empowered at the yoga centre, with Saturday classes being for women and their partners. As important as the telling of the stories and sharing of open information is for women, it is equally so for their partners, so that they can support and assist a woman in labour in an informed way.

My other 'nitty-gritty' birth education as to what the birth experience might be like came from my midwife, Mary Murphy. The wonderful thing about having a homebirth midwife is the continuity of care that you receive. I saw Mary once a month in the early stages of pregnancy, and towards the end it was every week and sometimes twice a week if she was in my area. As well as having a midwife who came to my home, I also had a doctor who I saw every two months. Between the two of them I felt like I was in great hands. They answered all of my questions without any hesitation or judgement and really made me feel this was my birth right from the start of conception to the birthday, which of course it was. It did take me a while to realise that this experience was my responsibility and no one else's.

During my first pregnancy I was teaching two pregnancy aquatic exercise classes, as well as general and deep-water aqua-fitness classes. I considered myself to be completely fit and healthy. Being fit enables the pregnant body to physically cope with the added stresses of carrying the extra weight from the baby and extra blood supply and fluid within the body. It can also assist in keeping the aches and pains away from the lower back, where many pregnant women feel weak and have dull pain due to the lower back hyper-extending to compensate for the increase in size and weight distribution at the front of the body.

For my second and third pregnancies I was still teaching aqua- fitness classes to keep in shape physically. I did even less reading to mentally prepare. Again, my knowledge came from having an inner belief and trust that everything was going to be OK with the birth and afterwards. Again, I attended yoga at the Family Nurturing Centre to exercise and stretch my body, and to share again the stories on the mats. This was my means of preparing in the most positive way possible. I was not interested in talking to strangers in the street or in the shopping centre about their experiences – where the tendency is often to debrief and dump on a pregnant woman – or attend hospital-based childbirth educational classes to learn about the hospital-based information, or attending groups of any kind for that matter. I knew what I wanted and could not be bothered defending or justifying my birth choice of water-birthing at home. During my first pregnancy I realised the value of sitting and listening to women talking about their positive birth experiences.

Maybe this is what women need most of all – an opportunity to talk in a room with other pregnant women and throw around ideas and simply connect with one another. After all, isn't that what women have done throughout centuries, around the world? Anita Diamant writes about this in her book *The Red Tent*, which I think is a wonderful book to read as it refers to a time in history when women would menstruate around the full moon together and spend this time in the Red Tent sharing stories of labour, birth, marriage and relationships.

Your Preparation – Choosing Childbirth Education That Suits Your Needs

Over the years, on countless occasions I have heard about the disappointment women and their partners have felt after attending antenatal classes facilitated by a hospital. The main concern has been that people felt they were all sitting facing the front of the classroom being formally taught the information as if in school, with very little emphasis on experiencing first-hand through interaction and sharing with others. In the hospital classes there is usually very little time for questioning or interaction with other couples attending, and little or no positive birth stories from women who have already birthed.

Couples have felt really disempowered, with classes that focus upon the need for women to have intervention and drugs, with little discussion of natural pain-relief techniques or choices. When educators were asked why they gave priority to teaching about the interventions in childbirth they reply along these lines: 'This is what the hospital advocates, therefore as educators we have to instruct couples about what this institution's policies are and what the doctors here want couples to know. This ensures the institution's point of view is understood.'

The idea of attending antenatal classes based on one side of the story is unfair and very disempowering for women and their partners. How can women learn to trust their body and prepare for birth in a positive way when fear itself is coming from within the hospital system?

Couples that have attended independent childbirth educational classes and then go along to classes run by the hospital are always amazed at how little emphasis is placed on the really important information and knowledge that empowers couples not to be afraid. These classes show couples how they can work together to cope, using natural and easy techniques that assist in diminishing the pain or intensity to a degree.

Like all classes, some attendees know very little about the actual birth, while others might have amazing knowledge and understanding through having read everything in sight. Those that have read a lot of books find they are often challenged or asked to be quiet if they ask too many question relating to child birth. I actually believe that some educators feel threatened when couples are well-read and educated and really know their stuff. This, of course, can 'upset the apple cart' and change the whole dynamics of the classroom setting, not to mention chew up the time. However, is having educated, well-read participants in an antenatal class such a bad thing? I think not.

As an independent childbirth educator, I believe it is fundamentally important to teach women and their partners everything about birth so that she/they will then be able to make suitable choices based on their knowledge. To do otherwise is cheating women and their partners of their right to really understand the intricacies of labour and birth. For this reason I strive to teach and share a broader and far more holistic approach to birth. Every childbirth educator needs to be accountable for the whole story being told, and not just a medical scenario of birth being taught as the 'norm'.

I guess the moral of the story is to choose your childbirth education classes very carefully. Paying out money for an independent childbirth educational class may assist you in receiving the broadest childbirth education there is, thereby ensuring that both you and the baby come through the labour and birth experience in the most natural and normal way possible. The value of this investment is priceless – how could anyone not even consider this a priority.

If you do decide on attending a hospital-based class, go with an open mind. They do, after all, have to teach according to the hospital's policies. This often doesn't lend itself to the holistic, more open approach to childbirth. To cover all bases a combination of both types of classes is recommended, so you arrive at your baby's birthday educated and knowledgeable about the type of birth experience you want to have, knowing full well what the hospital will allow and require from you.

4

You Have Many Options

Considerations When Planning
The Big Birth-Day

When I planned for each of my three births I had an idea in mind of exactly what I wanted during my labour. I developed my ideas through talking to my midwife, doctor and other women who had experienced water births, as well as through my exposure to Michel Odent's films. I had also seen Estelle's collection of videos that showed *beautiful births*, so I had a fairly good idea of what labour and birth looked like. With all of this input it was quite easy to draw upon this information and know exactly what I wanted. I had certainly seen and heard a little of what I didn't want, and that stood as a gauge to assist me in planning my unique birth experiences.

By integrating and connecting the mind and the body, and by taking fear out of the equation, a woman can allow herself to open up physically while mentally staying strong and focused. She can remain determined on many levels, overriding the need to throw in the towel and give up on her quest for a natural birth experience. Having a strong inner belief and trust in your body can help your body to birth in a very open manner. This understanding and concept is fundamental to natural birth.

Getting to this place starts with addressing what a woman wants and does not want when preparing for the labour and birth. The searching for and identification of what your particular needs are can begin from the day of conception. The earlier a woman can start to think about the inevitable labour and birth experience, the better. It is my belief that childbirth education classes should be started a lot earlier in pregnancy to assist with really clarifying what type of birth you want to experience. You can then find a suitable care provider, not the other way around. I have heard women say, 'But how can I prepare for a birth when I don't know what to expect?' My answer is to listen to your intuition and hear what it is telling you. Be aware of how you feel about experiencing labour and childbirth pain, about epidurals and episiotomy. Be empowered enough to know that you have a right to choose exactly what you want and don't want to experience. Choose a care provider who is going to honour your decisions and choices and not talk you into something you don't really want.

The next thing to think about is your choice of care provider.

Obstetric Care – Too Common Today?

I want to spend some time here discussing obstetric care, as this is currently the most common choice made by Australian women. I often wonder if women are genuinely aware that there are alternatives to obstetric care, so at the end of this section I present several other options for pregnancy and birth.

I found the following definition interesting to note, as it can be taken a number of ways, including literally – it is from *Webster's New Collegiate Dictionary*: 'Obstetric, from the Latin word Obstare, 'to stand in the way' and to 'stand in front of'.

It is important to remember that it is *your* birth – and also *your* baby's birthright to come into the world as calmly and peacefully as possible. No one has the right to stand in your way, preventing you from achieving this by taking control so it no longer is your birth experience. Birth does not need to be seen as a big mystery that only the medical professionals know how to deal with. It is the most natural thing a woman's body can do, and the less the medical professionals and support people interfere with this natural process the more probability a woman has of having a natural birth. However, more and more it seems that obstetricians working from a medical model of birth do indeed end up taking over.

I believe giving birth requires ninety percent positive attitude and ten percent physical ability.

If you are choosing an obstetrician, find out about his policies and beliefs about birth. Ask him to tell you how he feels about natu- ral childbirth. You are looking for the answer, 'Yes, without drugs, if you so choose!' If an obstetrician tells you there is no point trying to be a martyr, then you can assume he does not strongly support natural labour or childbirth. If this is so, I would suggest you change to another obstetrician with a more positive outlook on natural birth, or seek out a birth centre or homebirth midwife, if your choice is to try to birth naturally. This is your right and choice and not some- thing that you should have to fight for!

A woman should never be made to feel that she has to stay with one obstetrician just because she has seen him on a few occasions, getting to know him and hopefully building rapport. Shop around; after all, you may be the one paying the big dollars to bring your baby into the world, so choose to spend your money wisely. Often your obstetrician won't even make it to the actual birth or, to ensure they do, they may offer to induce you early, which can lead to further interventions. Even if you aren't personally paying the dollars to have an obstetrician, consider if you really need this level of care, as obstetricians are primarily medical specialists that deal with difficult births. They work on a 'birth is risky' mindset, rather than a 'birth is normal' viewpoint.

Obstetric care is specialist care, make no mistake about that. Specialists by nature are trained to intervene and can sometimes do so when it is not always necessary; I believe obstetricians find it very hard to step back when they see a woman in the throes of labour. After all, this is what you have paid the money for, isn't it? However, their service could come at a higher price than you bargained for. Is it right to assume that the majority of women in our society need specialist care? Is it right to presume that there is going to be a problem with every birth that occurs in the hospital system? I think not.

Once you are on the road of intervention it is hard to get off – as it can lead to more and more interventions till it is no longer your labour experience. This is known as the cascade of intervention, which once in motion is very hard to stop.

Medical specialists such as obstetricians can assist women and their partners if and when the time comes, which is better than handing over all of your control to a specialist doctor from the outset, or being at the mercy of hospitals' agendas and policies. I suggest you think carefully before deciding. Ask yourself, would you go out and buy a car or a house with as little thought as some couples put into choosing the right care provider for their birthing needs? No, I don't think so. Take your time – all six months of it if you have to – and explore all your possibilities.

If you want to know whether you have a good obstetrician, talk to other women that have birthed with this person. As a general rule, if they are fully booked up you know he/she is popular. On your first visit ask him/her about their birthing philosophy. If he or she cannot look you in the eye and answer you honestly perhaps move on to another carer. After all, how can someone that delivers babies every day not have some type of philosophy about birth! These professionals need to be accountable for what they do and how they feel about birth, and this begins in their consultation room by being as honest as possible with the paying customer.

If you are reading this and thinking, yes, I still want to have the obstetrician that I have chosen, make sure you do some more homework. Find out in detail what your obstetrician prefers – do not fly blind! Many obstetricians have protocols that can be quite restrictive, especially if you are planning an active birth.

However, there can be situations when having an obstetrician is very valuable, in order to draw on their knowledge and experience. If a woman has a medical problem, for example if the placenta sits over the cervix, an obstetrician will be needed. But it is a shame when healthy, fit women with no apparent overriding medical problems request an obstetrician as their primary care provider.

I want to state that I am certainly not rejecting the obstetric avenue of care. However, I am suggesting that women need to become aware of what their rights and choices are, and the more educated you are about your choices the better chance you have of having a good birth experience. I advocate that you are at least given a choice with the way you want to plan and experience your birth when the time comes. A good obstetrician will respect your choices and aim to make your birth experience as positive for you as it can possibly be.

However, often women are pushed into having interventions, such as being induced, or having procedures such as regular internal examinations or monitoring throughout labour that are not always necessary. It is often only after the birth experience that a woman asks, 'Why was that or this necessary?' This can lead to a sense of disempowerment and disappointment as they feel they had no control of their own birth experience. Once again, I would like to reiterate that birthing is about choice, and having your choices respected.

Despite advocating for completely natural birth, I know that sometimes the way a woman chooses to birth may not go according to plan. This can be for many reasons and it is when obstetric care may be necessary, to make sure the wellbeing of the baby and mother are monitored carefully.

The sad thing about obstetric care is that often first-time pregnant, young, healthy, fit women get pushed around and led to believe that they are putting their baby at risk or themselves at risk by not doing exactly as the obstetrician suggests when it comes time to birth. Listening and following without questioning is truly a shame and often results in a birth the woman did not want; many women have told me they wished they had listened and asked more questions.

From my experience in talking to many women, the consensus is that many women/couples feel annoyed about how the birth of their baby went. It is not only women but their partners who recognise that often women are not honoured, empowered or supported enough by the medical staff, in the way they ought to be during the most vulnerable state their body could possibly be in. Let's face it, being naked and on the edge of your pain threshold, with your vagina open, puts you in a pretty vulnerable state. That needs to be honoured and respected above all else.

Other Care-Provider Options

If, having read this 'food for thought' information about obstetric care, you have decided to forego this alternative, there are many other choices and options available to you.

1. Midwifery care – outside the hospital

A community midwifery program provides midwifery care out- side a hospital environment. In Western Australia we are very privileged to have a government-sponsored birthing program, which provides free community midwives who attend homebirths for women in the Perth metropolitan area. Most people with a community midwife as their primary carer choose to birth at home. New Zealand and the Netherlands have similar programs whereby the government funds midwives to attend women birthing at home, recognising that keeping the beds free in the hospitals ultimately saves the government hundreds of thousands of dollars every year. And, of course, recognising the many benefits for women that come from birth- ing in their own homes.

Going into labour empowered, well-educated and believing in your body can do wonders for your labour journey.

The Community Midwifery Program in Perth allocates a midwife to pregnant women who contact the service. (Of course, this assumes that pregnant women are aware that this program provides a midwifery service, which in our current culture is often not so!) The primary philosophy of the Community Midwifery Program is that pregnant women who experience ongoing, one-to-one midwifery care from a known midwife during their pregnancy usually have the best birthing outcomes – safe and woman-centered. Women on this program also have a doctor available as a backup care provider, should they need to transfer to hospital.

Other states in Australia are looking at running similar community midwifery programs based on this approach, where the midwife is the primary care provider. This type of care is chosen by seventy per cent of women in New Zealand.

2. Private homebirth

Women in Australia can also hire a midwife of their choice privately, usually with a planned homebirth in mind. I have already described homebirthing with a private midwife, as I did with my three children. Some medical funds in this country will cover a large percentage of the fee for having a private midwife. I definitely recommend this type of choice, but I am very biased in my opinion! To find a private midwife you simply look in the yellow pages. You can also contact a local pregnancy resource centre or women's health centre as these centres should be able to refer you to private midwives working in your area.

3. Birthing centres

I do understand that homebirth is not for everyone, and going to a birthing centre is a really good compromise if you feel that you want the best chance at a natural birth but do not want to birth in your own home. A birthing centre resembles a four-star hotel room with double bed, en suite bathroom and bath. Women are looked after by a team of midwives, all of whom the woman has met during her pregnancy. When a woman goes into labour any two of these midwives will be at her side to assist in the birth of her baby. In my experience, midwives at birthing centres are very supportive of natural childbirth and well-trained in focusing on the needs of a labouring woman and her support person/partner. They are also very experienced with natural childbirth as they see this on a daily basis and can assist first-time couples to feel completely at ease and reassured about the labour and birth.

The downside to this type of care is that the rules for admitting a woman to a birthing centre require you to be 'a picture of health', with no medical problems or conditions or previous problems during childbirth. The baby must also have no apparent problems or conditions in utero. The upside is that a woman gets to labour actively, moving about wherever she wants to go. Pain relief from drugs is often not available, but instead the option of using natural pain-relieving techniques is suggested and encouraged. However, should a woman feel the need to have pain relief, or if genuine complications develop, most birthing centres are attached to a main hospital, which makes a transfer quite simple if required.

4. Maternity units in public hospitals

Another birthing choice is to go to a public hospital and be admitted through the clinic. With this option, a woman visits the midwifery clinic at the hospital of her choice. Clinic visits occur once a month and a pregnant woman will also visit her GP on a shared-care basis. During the clinic checkups the midwife on duty will do all the usual pregnancy checks.

With this type of care, couples do not usually meet the midwives that work on the labour ward. So this could be considered a disadvantage, as it really is luck of the draw as to who you have assisting you on the birthday. Some research suggests that this 'lack of continuity of care' is an issue which can affect the birthing outcome, although a woman's antenatal notes are passed on to the labour ward so the ward midwives have a record of how your pregnancy has gone, an overview of who you are and any other relevant information. However, come birth-day you may not know or feel comfortable with the midwives on duty in the labour ward when you arrive needing support and encouragement.

If you choose this option, it is a good idea to do two things that will help to ensure you have the type of birth you have chosen, rather than being 'pushed around' by the hospital policies:

- Take in a really specific birth plan and put it up on the wall for all to see. An A3 sheet of paper with big writing on it will do the job!
- Take in a birth support person who really knows what birth is about and what the policies and procedures are, so that they can be an advocate for your birth plan. A birth assistant or 'doula' is perfect for this type of birth situation, as well as your partner. I have included a chapter on the role of a professional 'doula' in another section of this book.

5
It's Never Too Early To Plan!

It is so important for women to start thinking about the birthday as soon as they are over the first trimester of pregnancy. The overview I have included below highlights some of the more important aspects of planning, some of which could be thought about during the early stages of pregnancy. What is important to note is how a woman really feels about planning for the birthday, and giving lots of time and commitment to researching available options. The earlier this work is done, the more focused and clear women seem to be when the birth-day arrives.

Planning for your birth experience

There are many options and possibilities when planning your labour and birth, but first and foremost remember that this is your birth and no one else's. With that in mind, it is important not to prepare a guideline for birth based on what your husband, mother, sister or best friend wants to see. This is truly about you and your body and the way you feel you would like to bring your baby into the world. It is therefore imperative that you have a clear picture of what you really want. Going into the birth process with a clear understanding can and will help you to be prepared both mentally and physically. Birth, after all, is ninety per cent mental and ten per cent physical.

There are a number of ways to gain information and understanding of the types of births available, including attending antenatal classes, either hospital or private, reading books, watching videos and talking to other women about their positive experiences. Try to get to know yourself and look at what your needs are. Being pregnant can be one of the most wonderful times of looking at your life and all that has gone on before this moment. It is also a time of contemplation and planning for the future on many levels. As well, it may be a time of surrendering and letting go of many past beliefs and values. Take a look at how you really feel about birth, write down in a journal the many thoughts and feelings that may be coming up for you. Think about where your fears may lie, what is it that you are scared of? When fears come up, seek out someone to talk with to address these issues, as the more you talk over and look at this fear the quicker it can dissolve and melt away.

If women do go into labour in fear, it really can get in the way and ultimately affect the outcome of the birth. I have written about this very topic at length, quoting from Dr Grantly Dick- Read, in Chapter 10. Fear causes tension, which causes a height- ened sense of pain. This is why it is important to clean the slate and enter into childbirth with a clear consciousness. Know exactly what you want and don't want during your experience.

Below is a list of possibilities that you might wish to consider. I suggest that you read through them all and then choose the ones that you feel you would really like. A nice idea is to transfer these

Empowered Birth

onto a big A3 piece of paper to take with you to the hospital, or if homebirthing then hang in view for all to see. Above all, make sure you have discussed with your support people exactly what you want so they can assist you in the best possible way.

When planning your guideline THINK POSITIVE. Assume that there are not going to be any overriding medical complication occurring. However, should you feel locked into or totally committed to your birth plan, write on the back of your birth plan the following:

Sometimes the unexpected can happen. Should my baby or I be in any way in need of medical assistance and intervention I am open and willing to totally renegotiate my birth plan in order that the baby and I are under no undue stress or harm.

This is a good mantra to have as an underlying part of your birth plan, and it can help prevent the feeling of having failed should you need to have intervention or assistance in any form when you don't really want to but need to for you and/or your baby.

When planning your birth experience it is helpful to consider the following points:

1. Who would you like as your primary caregiver?
- Independent midwife
- Hospital-based midwife
- General practitioner
- Obstetrician
- Shared-care GP/midwife

2. Where do you want to birth?
- Home Birth centre

- Local hospital
- High-tech hospital

3. Who will be your support people?
- Husband/partner
- Sister
- Mother
- Friend
- Doula

4. Where will you seek your birth education?
- Books
- Yoga classes
- Antenatal aqua classes
- Private antenatal classes
- Hospital-based antenatal classes Videos
- Other women (friends, family, local shop assistant)

During Your Labour – Possibilities To Consider

- Make your birthing space as comfortable as possible, dim the lights, burn candles, incense or oil, sit on or lean over a fitball, use aromatherapy oils on your skin, have a massage on the lower back with oils, use heat packs on the pubic area and lower back.

- Have Bach Flower Rescue Remedy (or Australian Bush Flower Emergency Essence) to hand – this is a natural flower combination liquid given orally to assist a woman to stay calm and relaxed throughout her labour.

- Will you be naked?

- Will you wear clothes of your choice?

- Have you chosen a person(s) to be present at all times?
- Will siblings to be present throughout or for the delivery?
- Do you want to be able to remain active and move about and not just lie on the bed?
- Do you want foetal monitoring only when necessary (usually every hour), so you can move about freely as you wish
- Can you have foetal monitoring with hand-held monitor only so you can remain active and not be continuously strapped to a machine.
- If you're not in established labour will you want to return home/stay home?
- Food/fluids given when requested throughout the labour; it is not a bad idea to pack a lunch box full of all sorts of food you may want to snack on.
- Freedom to choose positions and activity in labour (walking, sitting, squatting, kneeling, sitting on fitball, leaning over a beanbag or fitball).
- Vaginal exam for specific medical indications only. (The right to say I do/do not want to know how dilated I am, the right to request number of dilation only – refer to Chapter 20, 'What do you do when labour starts', page 188, regarding this suggestion.)
- Full explanation of the risks and reasons why each suggested medical procedure is necessary. (Be informed, and if it doesn't feel right to you say 'no' or 'I need more time to con- sider that possibility – please give me five minutes to discuss that option with my support people/person.')
- Artificial rupture of the membranes. This is not always necessary, however if they are bulging I suggest you go for it.

- Artificial hormone (oxytocin) to boost contractions or induce labour will often be given in a drip, which means from that moment on you are attached to a bag of fluid. (Note: synthetic syntocin/oxytocin can be very intense and difficult for the body to handle and often leads to more intervention due to the severity of the contractions.)
- Access to a water tub or shower for natural pain relief – this is a fantastic way to take the edge off each contraction and enable your body to relax.
- Pain relief given only when asked for by the woman in labour. (Refer to Chapter 16, page 157, where I cover the advantages and disadvantages of the various types of pain relief.)

During The Birth Of Your Baby, Have You Considered ...

- Presence of partner, or persons to be present at the birth?
- Siblings to be present for birth?
- Position for second stage (the birth) to be decided by you?
- No specific time limit on second stage of labour if progress being made (some hospitals have a time limit of two hours)?
- Do you wish to have your perineum left to stretch naturally (if it is going to) or would you prefer to have an episiotomy (cut to the tissue between your perineum and your anus)?
- Would you like the midwife or birth attendant to assist the perineum to stretch as the baby is crowning to help it open more naturally by applying hot compresses and oil?

- Freedom to touch the baby during the birth?
- Mirror to be available to see what is going on?
- Father to assist in the birth by having a hands-on approach?
- Baby to take first breaths unassisted (no immediate suctioning)?
- Cord to stop pulsating before cutting – it can be felt by the mother to see if it has stopped pulsating?
- Immediate skin-to-skin contact with mother as soon as baby is delivered fully?
- You and the father/partner to discover the sex of the baby together, without anyone letting you in on the big surprise (Applies both to births where you have been told the sex of the baby and particularly if you don't know the sex!)?
- Oxytocin to be given as a needle in the thigh to help expel and deliver the placenta?
- If no oxytocin wanted, a physiological third stage to take place, and no injection to be given unless there is a sign of bleeding excessively?
- Baby on the breast immediately to help release the placenta, and to bond?
- Placenta to put in container and kept for you to take home?
- Vernix left on the baby and not wiped off the skin?
- Baby weighed and measured after initial bonding period and when first initial breast feed has occurred?
- Food and drink of choice given to mum on request?
- Dad/partner to bond with baby as soon as possible, holding, cuddling, etc.?

It Is Never Too Early To Plan!

Points To Consider After Your Baby Has Been Born

- Baby to remain with mother at all times (nights included)?
- Person of choice to be in your room/home when you need?
- Breastfeeding on demand from birth?
- Cabbage leaves ready for when milk comes in on day three?
- Lactation consultant to be called if assistance is needed with breastfeeding?
- Vitamin K for baby to be given orally/by injection, or not?
- Choice of what to do with your placenta?
- Nomination of person to phone family and friends with the wonderful news?
- Decide which day family and friends can start to visit (day four is advisable)?
- When and by whom do you want your baby bathed, if at all, in hospital?

Emergency Provisions And Considerations

- In the case of a C-section I would like my partner or support person to be present. (In most hospitals now only one person is allowed in the emergency department.)
- I will opt for an epidural as the form of pain relief for this procedure.
- When the baby is out I would like him/her to be placed on my chest, skin to skin.
- Should the baby need to go over to the baby warmer for further examination I would like my partner to attend to the baby.

- I would like to be able to see the baby at all times.
- I would like breastfeeding to occur as soon as possible and within the hour of birth.

Share your birth plan

Should you wish to discuss your birth plan with someone other than your primary care provider, a childbirth educator or doula would be suitable. There are many private childbirth educators and doulas who help women and their partners to prepare for their birth experience in this way, offering realistic and unbiased positive information. Feedback regarding a birth plan should be sought so you have someone to tell you if your approach to birth is realistic and likely to help you achieve your wants, needs and desires.

6

Having Siblings Present

My birth experience with a sibling present

From my experience, having my daughter Jaeosha at both of my sons' births was ideal. It was perfect for her to be present. She was the best little helper any woman could ask for, and assisted me in so many ways throughout both birth experiences. Not only did she pat my brow with a wet flannel and tell me she loved me, she kissed me and let me know how excited she was that I was having a baby. There were times also when she sat back and gave me the space I required to just get on with the job of birthing. I remember distinctly with both births she demonstrated a strong ability and inner sense of knowing that what I was doing was really important and she did not pester me in any way.

Jaeosha was two years of age for the first birth and four years of age for the birth of her second brother. In preparing her for the births, I do recall having talked a lot about my tummy and what was inside. I also showed her lots of photos of women birthing babies so when she actually saw me birth she would remain calm and unafraid. I think being really open and honest about what is going to happen is very important. The act of birthing is such a wonderful and natural event that siblings can enjoy being a part of it if it feels right to have them present.

Benjamin, aged two, on the other hand, was a pain in the backside when I went into labour with Jarrad, as every time I had a contraction he became needy and wanted to be picked up and cuddled. I went into such strong contractions that I just did not have the strength or energy to reassure him that what was going on for me was perfectly natural. I would have loved to have Ben there at Jarrad's birth, but I realised that it was just not going to work out.

If you'd like to have siblings present at a birth you have to assess the situation as it unfolds and have some backup and support for them should they start acting up and not coping once you have gone into labour. It can be hard to predict just how toddlers and children are going to respond on the actual birth- day. Some reasons not to have siblings at a birth may be because you feel it may scare them seeing you in labour, that their presence at the birth may slow you down, or that the siblings may become demanding and needy with no one to really care for them. Reasons in favour of having siblings at a birth may include wanting to share a wonderful family moment, that you feel it would be a positive learning experience, or for the pure fact you would just like the sibling present on the birth-day.

Some Anecdotes

A birth that I attended as a support person started with a long journey in the car to the Family Birthing Centre. My friend's seventeen-month-old boy was in his car seat watching wide-eyed as his mother laboured away making all types of noises and sounds. When we finally arrived at the Birth Centre he was ushered into the birthing room where he sat with his dad on the bed while mum laboured away. He looked adorable and calm with nothing but a quiet and content demeanour. When his baby brother was born his little face lit up, he was so happy to meet his brother at last. An explanation for his calm, contented state may have been due to the time when his baby brother was born. The birth took place around 1 a.m. in the morning and the little boy had been woken up from his sleep state earlier on in the night to come to the hospital. Regardless of the situation he truly looked like he enjoyed the experience, in awe of his mummy giving birth on the floor in front of him.

Another wonderful story I would like to share is from a lady whose three teenage sons attended her birth at home with a midwife present. As she explained, 'They could not do enough to assist me, with back massage, giving water and food, even holding the mirror so I could see the baby coming out, that was pretty wild.' The boys even assisted the midwife as the baby was born. Both the father and the boys caught the baby. When I asked this woman, 'How did you feel about the boys' close involvement in the birth?', she replied, 'I was overjoyed that they were interested and cared enough to be present and offer the support that they did, it surprised me really.' It also totally blew the boys away, the whole birth thing, and made them think about having protected sex as the thought of creating something so small and helpless made them realise that they need to be responsible for their own actions!

In summary

The main point I am making about siblings at births is that it is totally the woman and her partner's choice to decide if it is what they want. There can be situations where the best-made plans will not work out and a backup carer will need to be called in to take the siblings to another room or place. There can be times when having a sibling present works out to be a wonderful experience for everyone, even if there may have been initial doubts.

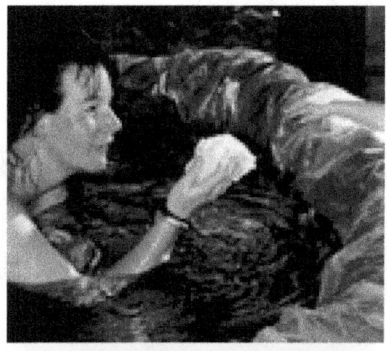

The homebirth environment is more conducive for siblings to be present during a birth, as when they get bored or tired they can just retreat to their bedroom or

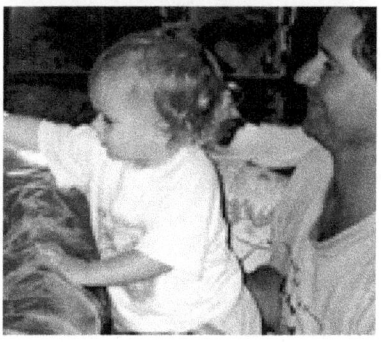

another part of the house. Being in the hospital or birth-centre environment can make it a little more difficult as often there is nowhere appropriate for children to go when they need a break from the birthing room.

It is usually best to allocate a support person who can specifically look after your older children if you wish them to be present for the birth. This ensures that the labouring mother can totally let go of the responsibility for her older children while she surrenders herself to birthing the new sibling.

7

Preparing For Your Marathon or Sprint

From my experience of working with women, I find that the ones who do exceptionally well giving birth naturally are those who have been preparing, not just mentally but physically by exercising throughout pregnancy. In particular, those who have been actively participating in sports and cardio type activities in the years leading up to pregnancy, and women who have participated in endurance-type events where they have really been challenged mentally and physically, do well in labour. Labour, after all, is like an endurance event for some women, like running a marathon or half marathon as the case may be while other women have a quick sprint to the finish line. The emotions, thoughts and feelings a person participating in an endurance event goes through are not that dissimilar to that of a woman in labour and why it is a great analogy that I like to use.

When I educate my clients and couples during my childbirth educational classes and sessions, I often refer to labour like preparing for a marathon running event. The diagram below demonstrates what I am referring to. Firstly, before you even begin the event, you need to make sure leading up to the big day that you are mentally and physically in great shape. I do not know of one single marathon runner who would not give 100% to their mental and physical preparation prior to running in an event, as should a pregnant woman preparing for her labour.

Make no mistake in labour your body is running a marathon on the inside even though from the outside looking at you—you look like you are 'in the zone' with the lights on and nobody home, all blissed out and oxytocinised up, just as you should be.

Secondly, before running a marathon you need to get as much rest as you can, eat nutritious and healthy food and have lots of water so you are really hydrated just as a marathon runner would.

This is the analogy of a marathon event that I use in my classes that represents the stages of labour and where a woman may be mentally and physically. Being a physical education teacher, exercise physiologist and long distance runner, I felt this was ideal to use as an analogy as it fits so well. I actually found myself in labour having to really dig deep mentally to stay focused within and just keep on going. It did take me back to when I was competing in cross country races and marathons, just how mentally strong and determined you need to be when competing and when in labour. The principles of what a runner and a woman in labour go through are so similar, particularly when looking at it in a diagram format with the stages of labour as you can see on the next page:

Excerpt from A Labour of Love II-Empowering through Knowledge to Create the Birth You Want and Desire.

I often use the analogy of a marathon to that of a labor. This diagram represents how often the two are very similar. The labor went from an 'intrinsic' response to labor to…gaby on your original outline of this page you wrote some more here but I can't read it! Can you send me an email with what you want to say?

The Labour Marathon

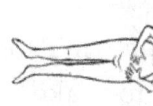

Warm Up Labour
- Period Cramping
- Feeling excited & nervous but happy it has started

Established Labour
- Hard work stage begins
- Need to focus within & work with dynamic rhythmical contractions

Transition
- Cervix is open
- Feelings of vunrability
- May have 'Hit the wall' with energy level
- Need to work hard to stay focused mentally & physically are nearly there!

Full Dilation / Pushing Baby Out
- Adrenalin kicks in & energy returns
- Get a 'second wind' as the end approaches - you at last
- Happy to meet your baby
- Feeling emotional & exhausted

Birth of Baby!
- Relief that it is over but feeling ecstatic

The Running Marathon

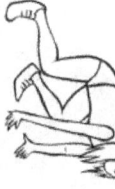

Warm Up Stage
- Warm up of muscles
- Feel nervous but excited
- Happy to have started

15km Mark
- Hard work stage begins
- Need to focus & find rhythm

35km Mark
- May have 'Hit the wall' with energy level
- Need to work hard to stay focused mentally & physically

40km Mark
- Adrenalin kicks in & energy returns have 'runner high'
- Get a second wind as the end approaches

Finish Line
- Relieved it is all over
- Ecstatic & happy you have completed your event
- Feeling emotional & exhausted!

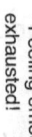

Thirdly, when the event begins, it does not matter how long it is going to take to run this marathon as time is irrelevant just as it is in labour. What is more important is that you get to the finish line having been strong, surrendering to the necessary sensations, staying positive, and feeling empowered and calm as your body performs as nature intended it to.

"Our task in birth is not so much to avoid the pain—which usually makes it worse—but to realise that giving birth is a peak bodily performance, for which our bodies are superbly designed."

Gentle Birth, Gentle Mothering: A Doctor's Guide to Natural Childbirth and Gentle Early Parenting Choices, Dr. Sarah J. Buckley

So, imagine now you are about to run your marathon/experience a labour. The warm-up phase of the event will see you moving from the start line to about the fifteen-kilometre mark. The time in which it takes you to get to this point does not matter. What matters is that you are surrendering and feeling really positive about what is happening to your body. This phase is where 'effacement' occurs. Effacement is where the cervix begins to thin out to paper-thin thickness, the wall of the birth canal gets thinner and the cervix changes shape and shortens.

The next phase is where you really begin to run your marathon and do some of the 'hard yards' work. This is often referred to as 'established' labour. This will take you from the fifteen-kilometre mark to the thirty five kilometre mark in any given time during your marathon/labour. Some women will do this in four hours, while some women may take over ten hours or more. Again, I want to stress that time is irrelevant and the time that it takes you to fully open your cervix through dilation is unique to you and each labour you experience. Like most long-distance events, one must watch out for 'hitting the wall' or 'burning out'. What

I mean by this is running out of steam and energy and feeling like you just can't go on.

Most marathon runners throughout the event need to replenish their fluids regularly by sipping small amounts often and drink energy glucose drinks and electrolytes to keep their blood sugar level and tissue salts up.. In labour, you have the advantage of being able to consume food if you wish, however just remember digestion is not the body's main priority when you are in labour. Most women can digest a small amount of low glycemic index (GI) foods which are ideal to keep her body fuel up. Further on in this chapter I have included a list of foods that you may consider eating during labour. Nature is so very kind to women in labour, as you will have opportunities in between your contractions to rest your body and close your eyes, drink, eat, pee, poo and ask for what you want if you wish to. It doesn't get more convenient than that, does it?

Limit your food intake—if you do eat too much your body will more than likely bring it all back up. Go easy on the amount, however, do not avoid food altogether for fear of throwing up! It is very normal to throw up during labour, just try not to aim it at your support people. Just recently, I was attending a birth and all I heard was, "I am…" and up and out it came all over me, the floor, bed and up the walls. It happens, it's Ok! On a more positive note, if you do throw up you contract your stomach muscles hard so that it causes you bear downwards with great force pushing your pelvic floor muscles which can assist the baby to move downwards.

Just to digress for a moment, here is a great alternative labour energy drink that can keep you going throughout labour just as if you were a marathon runner doing an event:

Labour-Aid

- 1 cup of coconut water
- Hydralyte powder
- Schuessler Tissue Salts by Martin and Pleasance
- 1 calcium tablet crushed and 1 magnesium tablet crushed

or

- 2 tablespoons of Musclease powder or a good quality Magnesium powder from the health shop mix with water —yum!

This combination will give you energy, hydration, and should prevent cramping of your calf and leg muscles, and keep your uterine muscles contracting effectively for any length of time needed.

When you near the thirty five kilometre mark, this is around the time you hit 'transition'. Just as the runner feels like he/she has hit the wall, you too may feel like you just can't go on. This phase is often characterised by women stating out loud how they just 'can't do it', or then begin to swear using 'Shit' and 'Fuck' words as that has the most impact for the woman to express herself and for those listening. It is a time of change and movement from the very nice 'passive hormonal labour state' of oxytocin—the feel good/love hormone and endorphins (nature's relaxant and peace maker)—to that of pure adrenalin to help you get the baby out of your body, wanting to push and bear downwards and give birth.

"You may feel like you go from experiencing a 'runner's high' to suddenly feeling like you have literally 'hit the wall' as everything is changing and

there is a certain vulnerability that goes with this change. Hang in there and stay strong, as before you know it you will feel the contractions in a different way."

Like the marathon runner, you may feel like you go from experiencing a 'runner's high' with all the wonderful opiates you have within you being released to suddenly feeling like you have literally 'hit the wall' as everything is changing and there is a certain vulnerability that goes with this change. Hang in there and stay strong, as before you know it you will feel the contractions in a different way. Like I did and most women do at some point, you will soon feel the baby's head moving down through the open cervix and often this comes with the strong urge to push. Just trust your body and have a little faith in yourself and your ability to keep on going. You have the choice to 'let go' of any inhibitions you may have and allow your body to just get on with the labour, staying out of your head thinking and analysing what you think is going on within you and just allow your body to do it.

Really allow the lioness within you to roar and make some noise. This can help prevent surrendering on running the final leg of your marathon course.

The transitional stage can go on from the thirty-five-kilometre mark until the forty-kilometre mark which I believe is when a woman is anywhere between seven centimetres to ten centimetres dilated, depending on where her baby is positioned and how fast a woman is dilating open. This is different for every woman, and is a rough estimate and guide only, and is purely my understanding and belief based on what I myself have experienced and seen as a doula of many different and unique birth occasions.

At the forty kilometre mark, a woman begins to push her baby down into the birth canal and just like the marathon runner at a world class event, she too is running with her arms up above her head as she enters the stadium, the crowd are upstanding and applauding this wonderful effort and journey from one place to another, and like magic she has energy and enthusiasm driven by adrenalin to just get on with the job at hand and birth, forgetting that she is tired and has had enough.

At the forty-two-kilometre mark and finish line, a woman receives her baby onto her chest and bonds with her baby as her support crew dance around doing the necessary tasks; begin celebrations and patiently await the arrival of the afterbirth/placenta. Like all good marathon events, the runner always finishes by having a good shower, big plate of food to energise and restore the body's fuel and drinks lots of water and sweet hot and cold drinks to get the blood glucose back up.

Women who are incredibly strong mentally and who have prepared themselves through exercise physically for this event—who are well informed and educated—do themselves a great favour. It really is about the preparation which makes a labour of difference!

Pregnancy And Exercise

It is important to choose an exercise program that is going to meet the pregnant woman's individual needs. If a woman becomes pregnant with little to no fitness, the ideal type of exercise program is one that maintains the pregnant woman's fitness level and does not try to increase it above and beyond the woman's capabilities. The heavy pregnant body needs to be treated with respect by its owner and by the fitness leader who is responsible for this specific population group. If a woman is going into pregnancy with great fitness, due to participating in regular types of fitness classes prior to conception, it is fine to continue with regular exercise until she personally feels too heavy and tired to continue and feels the need to slow down.

Benefits Of Exercise – Physical And Social

From my experience over 25 years of conducting specific antenatal aquatic exercise classes, including a deep-water running, toning/strength and aquatic relaxation classes in a hydrotherapy pool, there are many benefits for pregnant women. Participants often express how fantastic and positive, not only physically but mentally, the classes are, as they learn so much about their own body – how to work it, how to stretch it out, and how to nurture it.

During the classes there is always discussion about birth. I often share stories of the women in the class who have just graduated into motherhood (with their permission), this I know assists my clients to gain an understanding of what birth is all about, as the stories come from women they know, an authentic source of inspiration. And of course, most importantly, and especially in today's society, they make friendships and connections with other women in the same situation as themselves. As many women find, pregnancy is a time in their life when they want to connect with other women on many levels and an exercise class tailored to pregnancy enables this to occur in a non-threatening way.

By telling the birth stories of women who have just graduated from my aquatic classes I am able to share first-hand information that touches the women on a very deep level. (It serves well to not only inspire women, but it plants the seed that gives them the belief and trust around birth that they too can do this job their body is designed to do.) Subconsciously, women then go if Mary or Jane can give birth in such an amazing way so can I. The more stories they hear the more this concept and belief gets reinforced. It is a powerful way to assist women to gain empowerment around birth. Another powerful development that comes from these classes is an incredible bond is shared be-

Aquatic Exercise

Water exercise classes are ideal for women to attend when pregnant as the water totally supports the body, whether attending a chest-deep class (feet touching the bottom) or a deep-water class (totally suspended). There are many swimming pools around Australia that offer specific antenatal classes nowadays, as water is so conducive to exercise when pregnant. However, if a specific pregnancy class cannot be found, a general aqua-fitness class would be suitable, paying attention to the following conditions and problems pregnant women may experience physically when exercising in deep-water classes.

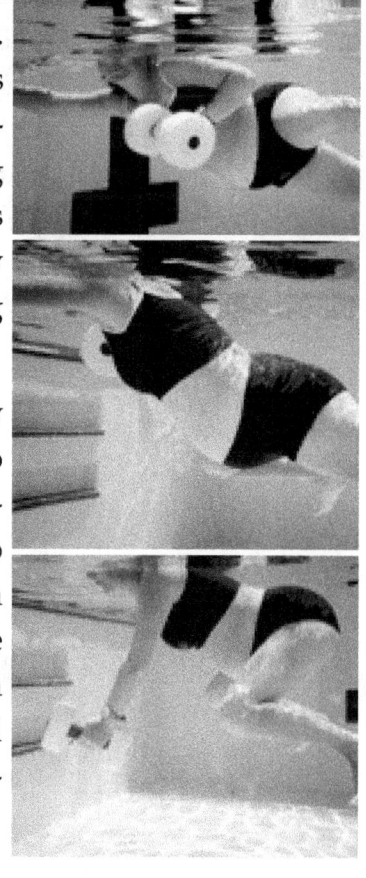

A word of warning: It is potentially dangerous for a pregnant woman to wear a buoyancy belt when participating in deep-water classes, due to the extreme pressure and restriction caused by where the belt sits on the body. The baby's supply of oxygen through the blood may be inhibited and restricted to the placentaand umbilical cord, when the mother is

tween these women, not only because they have been exercising alongside each other week after week, but because each woman shares a common goal and objective: a birth, which they know will inevitably occur.

Over the 25 years that I have run these classes amazing life long friendships were created as well as pregnancy support coffee catch ups and post birth Mum and bub groups.

One of the greatest things about a specific pregnancy class is that the graduates will often return within a few weeks to share first-hand their fantastic birth story. It is always fascinating to see the various reactions of the pregnant women, listening intently. Even with all the positive preparation around them they are always amazed when a woman comes back to the class and tells a wonderful account of a positive birth experience. Grantly Dick-Read expresses this so perfectly:

So firmly rooted throughout society is the belief that childbirth is a painful and frightful affair that even those who can state quite honestly, from their own personal experience, it is not so, are disbelieved and even laughed at.

Women can feel very isolated when they fall pregnant – some stop work and find that they are bored at home and tired all the time. A pregnancy exercise class can enable women to communicate their fears, troubles and stories in a supportive, non-judgmental way. And they can start to feel good about the changes that are taking place in their body as they realise others are experiencing the same feelings and sensations, both good and uncomfortable. Some may feel the need to just cry and let go of their emotions. It is not uncommon to feel emotional and teary at the drop of a hat!

immersed in the water and physically moving, with her heart rate elevated. A pregnant woman can still participate in deep-water exercise classes using other forms of hand-held buoyancy equipment as an alternative, to gain the extra buoyancy needed to execute the moves efficiently and effectively.

Walking

Walking is one of the best activities for fat-burning, especially if the walking is done at low to moderate intensity. One of the problems pregnant women often find, however, is that the bigger they grow the harder it is to walk longer distances. It is important to listen to and honour your body, and if walking becomes a task to be endured rather than an exercise that you enjoy, perhaps you may need to consider another more suitable form of exercise.

Types of yoga

Hatha yoga is a form of gentle yoga that enables pregnant women to stretch out their tired and aching muscles. It is ideal for those who have not participated in any form of yoga before. Other types of more vigorous yoga are Ashtanga and Ayurveda. Like all exercise regimes, if you have participated in yoga prior to falling pregnant, your body will be accustomed to exercising in a certain way. Hence, continuing on through your pregnancy should be suitable for you. For others starting out, a vigorous yoga style may not suit your needs. Do shop around, till you find a style that suits you. Yoga really is a wonderful way to tune into your body and ease any niggles or cramps that you may be experiencing.

The benefits of swimming

Swimming has many benefits for the pregnant body. Obviously the body is supported and free to move in any direction and is enabled by buoyancy to stay afloat. A person's fitness level can really be improved with swimming laps, as the action of overarm totally works the aerobic energy system, causing the heart to beat faster, the blood to pump more quickly and the body temperature to rise. The overarm or front-crawl action is the most suitable swimming stroke to perform, as it unilaterally works the body causing a dual positive muscular activity which balances the body structurally and in postural positioning.

Breaststroke is one that I recommend pregnant women stay away from. The leg action, which is a frog-kick movement, can exacerbate or create bad sciatica pain and can cause pubic stabbing pain. Both are conditions that pregnant women need to be aware of and try to avoid at all costs, as they really can become nasty and hinder movement substantially towards the final weeks of pregnancy.

Pregnancy fitball classes

Sitting on a fitball when pregnant and in labour is very relaxing as your bottom and thighs actually mould into the ball. The pressure and opening a woman experiences through her pelvis can feel very nice, not to mention the almost magical feeling of being massaged through the bottom and thighs when one rocks, rotates or softly bounces on the ball. A lot of the exercises that can be done on the ball are similar to pilates exercises. Pilates is a form of exercise that focuses on specific muscles and works at toning and strengthening weaker muscles by using specific movements.

Types of Cardio Classes

The cardio classes that I am referring to are the types of classes one can attend at a gym complex or at an F45 centre. Cardio classes like Les Mills are pre-choreographed classes to music which offers Body Jam, Step, Body Pump and New Balance classes, just to name a few. Free style functional fitness classes are not pre choreographed and comprise of weights, cardio moves, steps, boxes, fitballs, bands and rowing machines and bikes. Depending on your fitness it is quite suitable for pregnant women to continue participating in cardio/functional fitness classes, if that is the type of exercise their body is used to. As long as your body is accustomed to this style of exercising, you can continue. However, having said that, there will come a time when the body just feels too awkward, heavy and uncoordinated to want to continue, and listening to your body when that time comes is very important.

If you have never participated in any type of cardio class it may be wise to give this form of exercise a miss until after the birth and recovery period. The reason I suggest this is because the higher intensity moves can be too strenuous for non-pregnant newcomers, let alone a pregnant woman. Not only that, the relaxin hormone kicks in very early on in the pregnancy, which causes ligaments and muscles to become lax and pliable, hence there is a greater risk of injuring oneself. The last thing a pregnant woman needs is an injury, from exercising during thier pregnancy.

Cycling

The thought of getting on a bike while pregnant did absolutely nothing for me. In fact, I could not think of anything worse.

Personally, I found sitting on the seat very uncomfortable and it exacerbated my chronic sciatic pain. I even bought a gel seat to see if that would make a difference. It didn't. As I write these words, I look out the window to see my girlfriend riding on her bike, thirty weeks pregnant with number five. Her little boy looks amused and content in the seat on the back and her three gor- geous girls are in tow. I asked one day how she felt about being pregnant on the bike, and she calmly replied, 'It doesn't bother me at all, I love it, in fact that's how I get my exercise.' It is very individual as to what each pregnant body will be able to do in terms of physical exercise, so just tune in and see what suits your needs.

Exercises to avoid when participating in an exercise program

When participating in any type of fitness class, land or water, care is needed when executing abdominal exercises. Up to about fourteen weeks in pregnancy, it is safe to keep on training those muscles to brace and contract. After fourteen weeks, these muscles need to start relaxing and letting go. It is not uncommon for a woman who has tight, strong abdominal muscles to experience sharp ligament pain and abdominal stretching in the form of a dull ache around the uterus as it attempts to stretch in the second and third trimesters.

If lots of abdominal exercises are performed, with the legs coming into the chest, or lots of tuck jumps, or burpees with a crunch/curl type action, there is a strong possibility that the linea alba may split up to three to four centimetres wide. The linea alba is situated between the left and right rectus abdominis muscle group, starting just under the sternum and running vertically down to the pubis. When the linea alba splits this is known as diastesis recti; it is very common and not at all painful but feels terrible when touched, as all you can feel is a gaping hole where this tissue used to be joined together.

To avoid tearing and splitting the linea alba, consider stopping abdominal exercises after the fourteenth week of pregnancy. In order to prevent a tear you need to keep a watch on how you move your body. Try not to jackknife your body getting up and out of bed; instead, sit up with your legs straight. If you are at the swimming pool don't attempt to pull yourself up and out of the pool at the side, use the steps or ladder. Some women may do everything possible to prevent this split and a small one may still occur due to the amount of stress and force outwards during later stages of pregnancy, even if you have really watched your body movements.

Swimming is well-suited for the pregnant woman, but there are a few points to be aware of. As previously mentioned, breaststroke and the frog-kick should be avoided as this can aggravate a condition called sciatica. Sciatic pain is caused by excessive movement (due to the hormone relaxin) in the sacroiliac joint, putting stress and strain on the nerves running through and near this joint, the sciatic nerve being one. Women will often com- plain about a sharp stabbing pain at the back of the hip buttock area. The pain may also grab or refer down the leg, causing problems for some women when they walk or climb stairs.

To minimise sciatic pain, any form of abduction and adduction should be avoided at all costs. In plain English, taking the leg away from the midline of the body (imagine you have a vertical pole running from the tip of your head down to your feet, which are together) to the side and bringing it back in to the midline should be avoided. For example, a frog-kick rotates the hip joint in this exact manner, placing extra stress on the sacroiliac joint. Executing any inner and outer thigh exercises in aqua fitness classes, or in the gym during a circuit or during land- based aerobic classes, should be avoided.

Even some love-making positions can cause or aggravate pre-existing conditions, leaving a woman in a pretty dire predicament! I actually had a woman come to my class who told me she literally got stuck on top of her husband while they were making love. In a moment of passion there she was, screaming in acute sciatic pain, while her husband presumed it was the enjoyment of the occasion, made no comment, and continued like a real trouper, until she screamed at him to stop!

The moral of the story is try to keep your legs together and consider abstaining from sex if you are suffering from acute sciatic pain, as it could get worse. Something else I suggest to women is to keep your legs together when getting into and out of the car (sit on a plastic shopping bag and swivel) as this prevents pressure on the sacroiliac joint and pubic bone.

Symphysis pubis is another condition that can occur when a woman participates in a fitness program while pregnant. Like sciatica, this pain and sensation is caused by abduction and adduction, inner and outer thigh movements. Due to the presence of relaxin within the body, gravity pulling us down to the earth, the extra weight from the baby, fluid and increased uterus size, the pelvis may start to open. As the relaxin hormone increases month by month the pelvic bones move apart, and the baby drops down to wedge nicely in the correct birth position. This can result in the little fibrous band across the pubic bone pulling apart and snapping back, causing a sharp stabbing-type sensation, which from my own experience is really painful. Again, I want to highlight that not every woman will experience this, but not doing any extra inner and outer thigh exercises or unnecessary opening and crossing of the legs will reduce the likelihood of this problem occurring at all.

Yoga is ideal when pregnant, as it can stretch out the tired, aching muscles of the body. Yoga is wonderful for the simple fact that it helps to stretch the muscles of the entire body, especially the lower and upper back as well as the hamstrings (muscles down the back of the upper thigh). These muscles are often very tight when the lower back is under stress and strain from the extra weight at the front of the body.

One of the problems with carrying a baby internally on the front of the body is a woman's centre of gravity shifts down, causing the body to become unstable in balance. This is why some pregnant women fall over. The extra stress that is placed on the lower back, causing a swayback, is referred to as lordosis. Lordosis is an exaggeration of the lumbar curve of the vertebral column and is caused by the extra weight at the front of the body and weak erector spinae (lower back muscles). Yoga can greatly assist in strengthening and stretching these areas of the body.

Yoga stretches counterbalance the body. Where the lower back may be hyper-extended (swayback), a stretch leaning forward will assist these muscles in letting go and lengthening. Holding yoga poses also helps pregnant women to gain confidence in their balance once again and causes strong bracing of the internal postural muscles of the body. Abdominal bracing is one of the most important things to learn while pregnant. Correct abdominal bracing helps to keep the postural muscles strong, which can reduce or prevent the onset of lower back strain, weakness and back pain.

Bracing of the internal postural muscles can also occur while participating in aqua aerobics, fitball or just by sitting up straight in a chair. Abdominal bracing is basically demonstrating good posture, with emphasis on pulling your abdominal muscles in towards your backbone. Keeping a straight back is also imperative, whether you are sitting or standing.

Thoracic kyphosis, rounding of the shoulders, can be quite noticeable in pregnant women. This rounding of the upper back is due to the downward traction of the upper back and spine. Factors affecting this condition include an increase in breast size, poor posture, an unsupportive bra, or tight, weak pectoral (chest) muscles that may need strengthening and stretching. If a woman has noticeable lordosis the first thing that I suggest is that she gets fitted with a good bra at a maternity shop. In the long-term, extensive lordosis can eventually lead to severe headaches and neck pain, which can refer down the arms and back causing tingling, numbness and weakness. This is avoidable, and participating in a yoga class can prevent or eliminate this prob- lem within a few sessions.

The Pelvic-Floor Muscles

The pelvic floor is made up of lots of muscles that support your bladder, uterus and bowel. In order to keep these bands of muscles in shape, women need to contract and pull these bands up on a regular basis. The most effective way to work these muscles is to pull them up in three stages or 'floors'. I often recommend that women say to themselves as they pull up and tighten these muscles, 'first floor, second floor and third floor' – as if these muscles are a lift elevating up through a building. Be sure to hold the elevator at the third floor for as long as possible before coming back down to the ground floor.

Like any muscle in the body, the only way to increase its strength is to work it in repetitions and sets, for example by pulling up to the third floor six times with a thirty-second rest in between on the ground floor. Then have a minute's rest to let the muscle recover, before doing another six repetitions, with another minute's rest again afterwards, then a final six repetitions to finish. You would then have executed three sets of six exercises.

How far you lift and pull the muscles of the pelvic floor up into your body will very much depend on the strength of your muscles. The stronger the pelvic floor, the more dynamically you will be able to lift and pull these muscles in. The important thing to remember is to try not to pull your abdominal muscles into your backbone, as these muscles have no part to play in strengthening the pelvic floor.

Trying to visualise a figure-of-eight band of muscle fibres that incorporates the vagina and anus, lifting up towards the sky, will assist in feeling the right muscles being worked. Women need to tighten the pelvic-floor muscles and squeeze both the front (vagina) and back (anus) passages. An analogy I often suggest to women is to imagine half-inserting a tampon, then using your pelvic-floor muscles to squeeze the tampon all the way in to the vagina. This analogy gives a pretty good idea about the muscles needed to complete this task.

From my own personal experience, I have to suggest that just doing one pelvic-floor exercise at the traffic lights does not even get close to improving the tone and strength of this muscle group – you really do have to do sets and repetitions. Also, stopping the flow of urine can actually aggravate the urethra and pelvic-floor muscles and is not recommended by incontinence specialists.

Another successful method is to tighten up your muscles around your partner's penis during intercourse. By doing your exercises this way your partner can give you feedback as to whether a squeeze can be felt. If you do not have a partner, two fingers can be inserted into the vagina and you yourself can feel for the squeeze and tightening.

The best possible position for doing pelvic-floor exercises is in a seated position; however, they can be done lying on your side. The advantage of doing your pelvic-floor exercises in a seated position is that you work against gravity, hence your pull upwards may be more proficient and dynamic. Sitting on a fitball is really comfortable for doing pelvic-floor exercises, as is doing them in a hydrotherapy pool leaning up against the wall with your legs slightly bent.

8
Optimal Foetal Positioning Makes A Labour of Difference!

Any of my aqua-specific class participants will tell you what a stickler I have become for getting women to acknowledge where their baby is sitting inside their body and just what they can do to assist their baby into a favorable position for birth. This acknowledgement and push came after reading *Understanding and Teaching Optimal Foetal Positioning* by Jean Sutton and Pauline Scott who live and work in New Zealand. They suggest due to our Westernised/sedentary lifestyles, women are no longer leaning forward at all throughout their day due to not having to perform tasks and skills of manual labour around the house, like chopping wood or scrubbing the floors. The cause and effect being we are witnessing more and more babies being in a posterior position or OP (*Occipito Posterior*) as it is technically referred to, where the baby's spine is to the mother's spine and back of the pelvis.

Jean and Pauline, like myself, believe it is of utmost importance to get a baby into the optimal foetal position as early on in the pregnancy as thirty weeks, for this is when a baby is starting to rotate around and is settling into the pelvis in readiness to be born.

Having run aquatic and fitball pregnancy specific classes for many years, optimal foetal positioning was something I was always aware of and it was always at the back of my mind, however until I read *Understanding and Teaching Optimal Foetal Positioning*, I did not consciously tune in to just how important optimal foetal positioning is in relation to birthing outcomes. That wake up call came to me about 15 years ago when I was noticing so many women coming to me with posterior positioned babies who would literally endure these long hard drawn-out labours as their body tried to turn their baby with the contractions to the anterior position in labour, or they birthed their baby in a posterior facing position with intense back pain.

It is for this very reason that I now encourage women to do some fundamental activities from thirty weeks through to the baby's birth-day/night once they know they have a baby head down.

The three things I get women to do are what I call:

- Tummy time (between 30 to 40 plus weeks)
- Ball time (any time from 30 weeks onwards—when head is down in pelvis)
- Peri Prep time (from 35 weeks onwards—every third day until birth) this is covered thoroughly in chapter 22

Tummy Time

Firstly, I will focus and explain what tummy time is: Tummy time is about getting a woman to lean forward for twenty minutes a day two to three times a day if possible. This can be done incidentally while carrying out other tasks or on purpose in a desired place and position.

I find women can easily perform this task while:

- Talking on the phone—leaning over the kitchen table or bench top
- Watching TV—leaning over a fitball, bean bag or back of your arm chair or couch
- Swimming in the pool—in a prone (face-down) position with mask or snorkel (gravity is best though)
- Participating in a Yoga class—child pose, dog pose and cat pose
- Attending antenatal childbirth educational classes—sitting on a fitball, leaning over a fitball or beanbag (not sitting upright in an uncomfortable chair)
- Scrubbing and cleaning the floors—on your hands and knees (No, I am not kidding!)
- If on the computer, sit on a fitball or ergonomic chair that forces your body forward and back to be straight
- Playing on the floor on your hands and knees with your other children
- Pulling the weeds out of your garden or planting new plants in garden beds
- Chopping the firewood if you have a fireplace—some people still do!

Below is a picture of a woman leaning over on hands and knees:

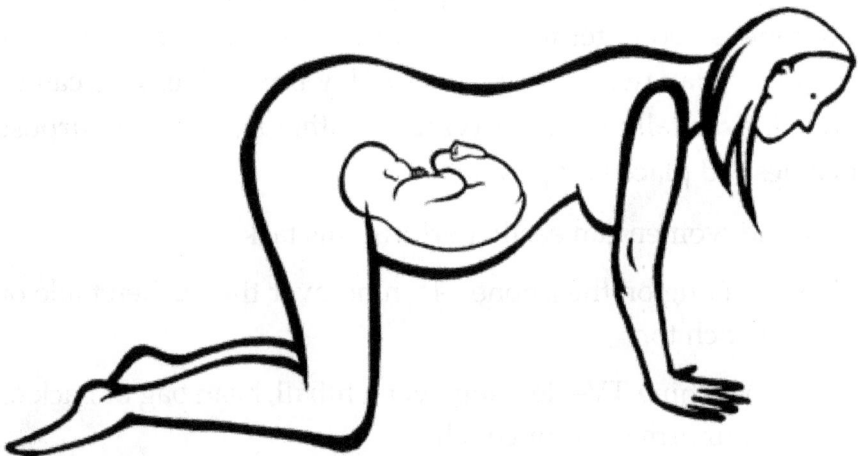

In order to rotate your baby to an anterior position or OA (*Occipito Anterior*) position as it is referred to, so that your baby may enter the pelvis with more ease, it is so important that from thirty weeks in your pregnancy, you avoid laying on your modular couch that has the 'chaise', or reclining chair such as a La-Z-Boy, as this really does interfere with what optimal foetal positioning is about. I know this can be very difficult and tempting when you are pregnant and feeling tired and heavy, and nowadays we have such comfortable furniture that looks like a bed and beckons us to come and lay on it in the dreaded reclined position. Avoid doing so at all costs—I really can't stress this enough! Ban yourself from lying down on this furniture for this very short time in your life. I know personally that all you really want to do is lay on that couch at the end of a day and rest, however laying on your back can rotate your baby into a posterior position which is not really conducive to a straightforward and easy birth. Labour with a posterior baby position is hard work, make no mistake about that. Women can birth a baby in a posterior position however, it is harder on the woman due to the intense back ache that does not go away when the contraction is on and off, and often the labour can be very long and hard. Women who do labour with a posterior positioned baby need a medal for being so strong with incredible endurance.

Below is a diagram of a posterior baby:

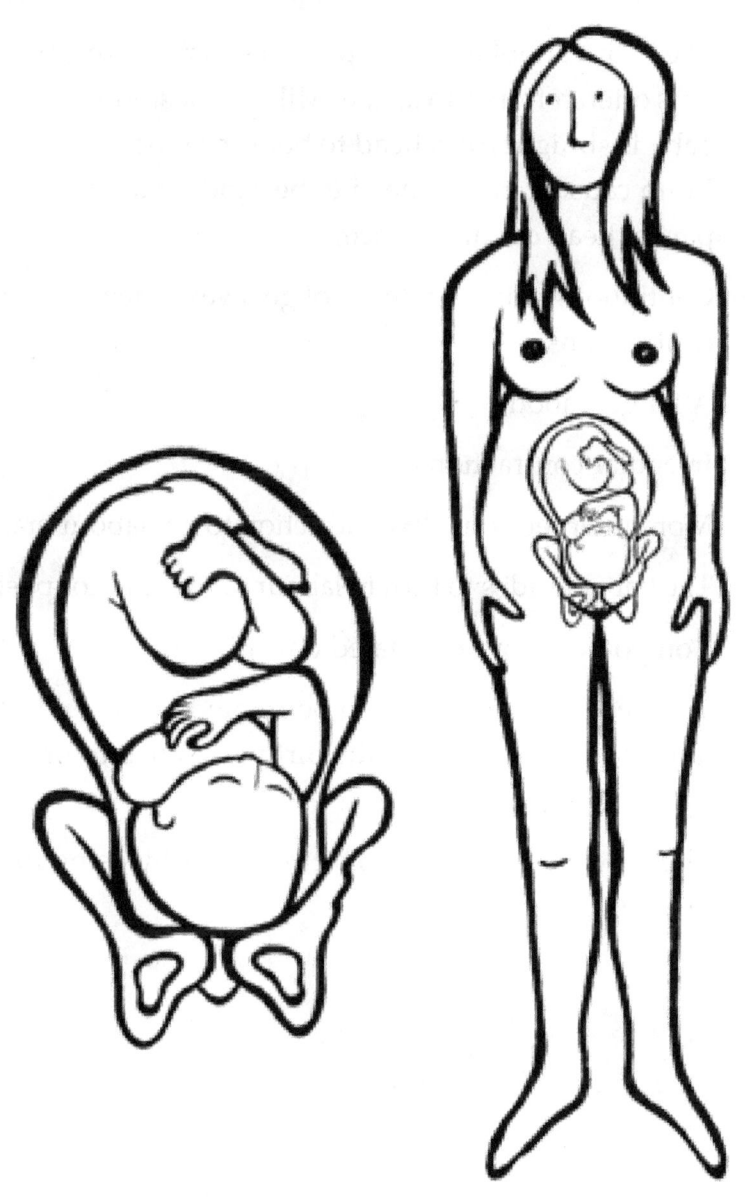

Having a baby in a posterior position may cause the following:

- Labour pain in your back/constant intense back ache that does not go away
- Pain deep in the pelvis and hips on one or both sides
- The baby cannot enter the pelvis as easily in this position (it is often referred to as the 'Military position' where the baby is straight from head to bottom spine to spine with Mum causing baby's head to be rigid presenting widest part of head circumference)
- Continuous pain that does not go away when in between contractions
- A longer labour
- Irregular contractions
- More interventions (like induction to get labour started)
- The baby decides to turn in labour to the anterior position
- You go over your estimated date of birth
- The need for your baby to be rotated at the end of the labour with the head in the birth canal using forceps or vacuum or both
- The need for assistance to birth your baby using forceps or vacuum

Below is a diagram of an anterior baby:

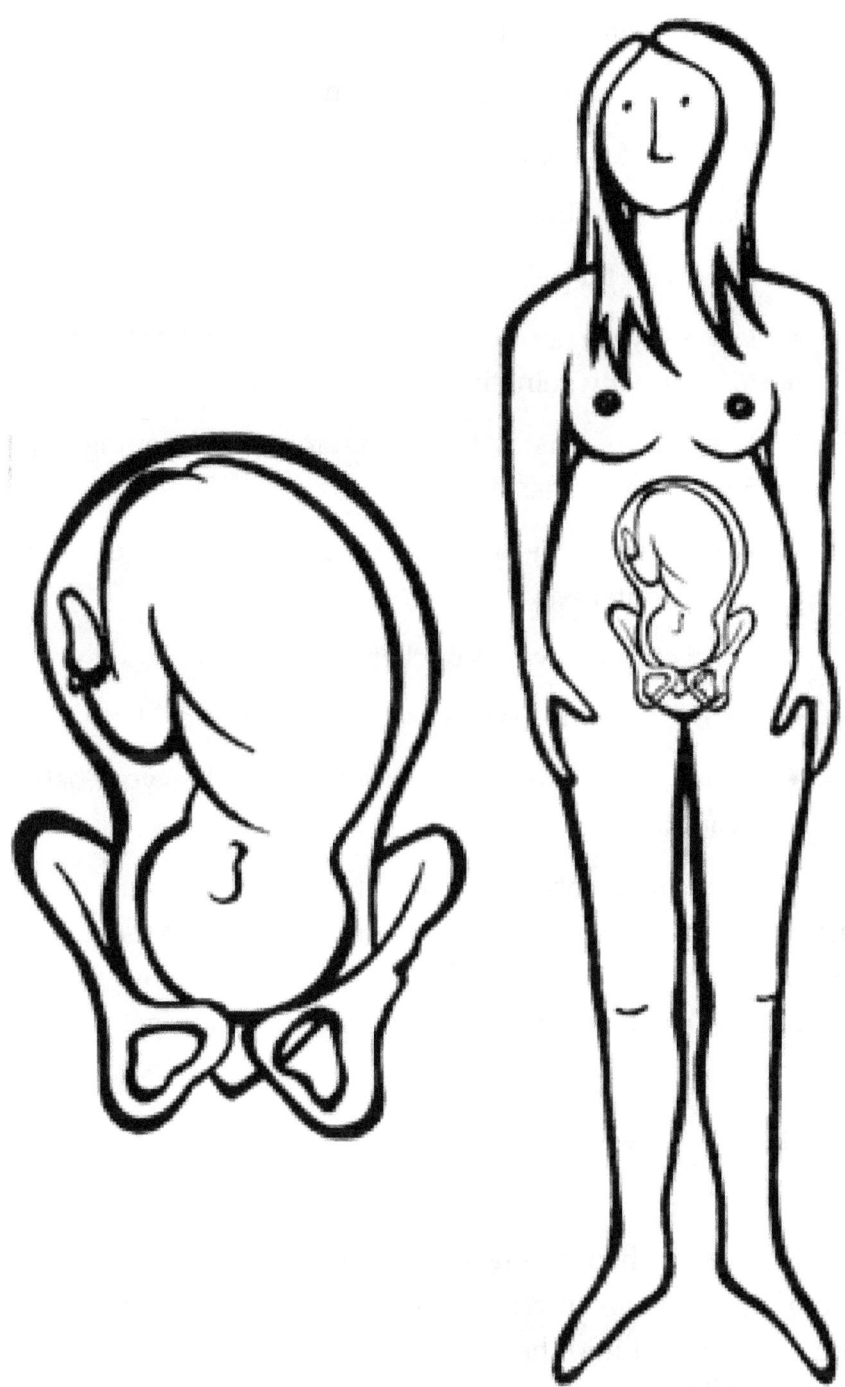

Having an anterior position baby may mean:

- Labour being shorter
- Less pain associated with labour
- You will receive rest periods in between contractions
- Baby may be born closer to estimated dates
- Less need for pain relief
- Less likely to need interventions at the end of labour due to your baby being in a better position
- In order to assist with optimal foetal positioning, try to avoid at all costs:
- Laying back in a semi-reclined position on furniture and in bed
- Long car trips with a bucket type seat
- Sitting with the legs crossed on any type of chair
- Squatting—should not be attempted unless your baby is head down or in an OA position

If you are still working up until your estimated date of birth try not to slouch on your chair at your desk—try to use an ergonomic chair that tilts forward or sit on a fitball. Below are some practical ideas that I encourage women to do to get the baby down into the pelvis.

Ball Time

Ball time is about getting on a fitball every day once you know your baby is in an anterior position to encourage your baby to head down and into the pelvis rim. If you don't have a fitball, go out and buy one as you can use it to labour on as well. Make sure when you sit on your ball that your knees are lower than your pelvis. Once your baby is in the anterior position, you have less chance of your baby deciding to rotate into an OP position or worse still, deciding to go breech!

Ball time is about sitting on your fitball for twenty minutes or more a day, while swinging and rocking your pelvis forward and back, side to side, doing big round circles one way and back the other way. Then I often suggest you pretend to write your name on the floor with your vagina in cursive writing (this is always interesting and very entertaining in a class!). You can finish with your pelvic floor strengthening exercises (squeezing your pelvic floor muscles up to the 1st floor, 2nd floor and 3rd floor and holding for the count of six, and then letting it down slowly. This can be repeated eight times over, having a minute's rest and repeating two more times. All up, you are doing three sets of eight exercises).

If you are having bad problems with peeing when laughing, sneezing, chasing your toddlers around or jumping up and down when exercising then you will need to do three sets of eight three times per day to really get these muscles to engage and become strong once again. The more you do the exercises the stronger your muscles will become the less likely you are to leak urine and have a little accident. Remember if you go into labour with strong pelvic floor muscles your recovery after will be so much better and some women actually have great strength straight away post-birth because of all the effort they put in prior to birth.

The thing to ask yourself is how strong are my pelvic floor muscles and how open is my pelvis?

Many women I work with have terrible pelvic floor muscles and very tight ligaments around the pelvis even though they have the wonderful 'relaxin' hormone in their body that should be assisting with ligament laxity in their pelvis. As for the pelvic floor muscles, women seem to think that the stronger the pelvic floor muscles, the harder it is to push a baby out. This is completely wrong and contrary to popular belief is in fact the opposite. The stronger the pelvic floor muscles, the easier and more dynamic the pushing can be, hence the pushing/birth phase of a labour can go very quickly.

Some of ways to open the pelvis are as follows:

Yoga positions such as the Angel/Child pose as shown below

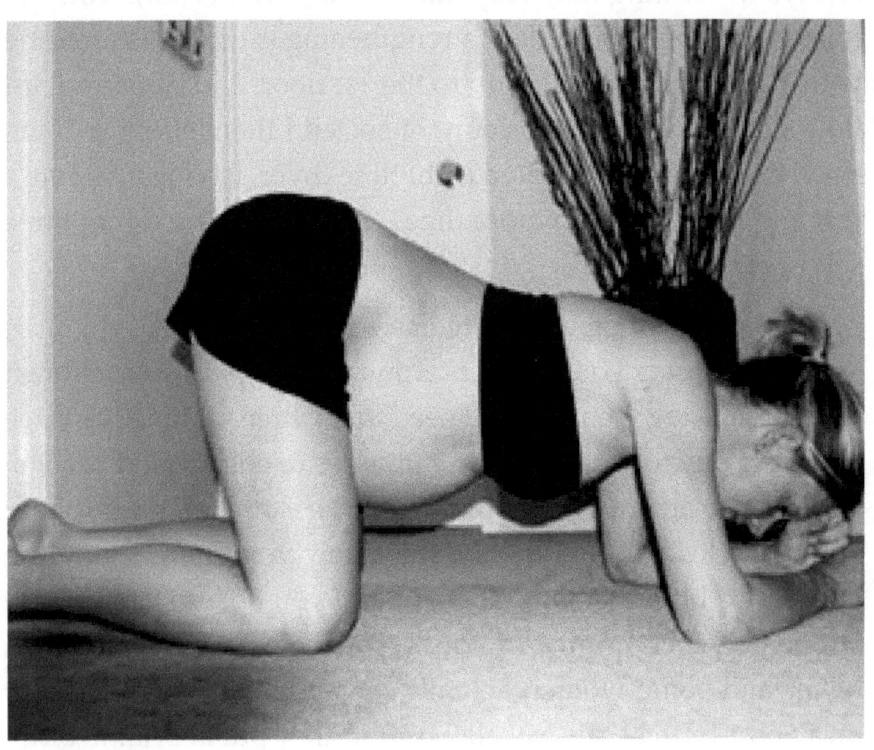

Kneel with one leg up rocking through your pelvis and then change to the other leg as seen below

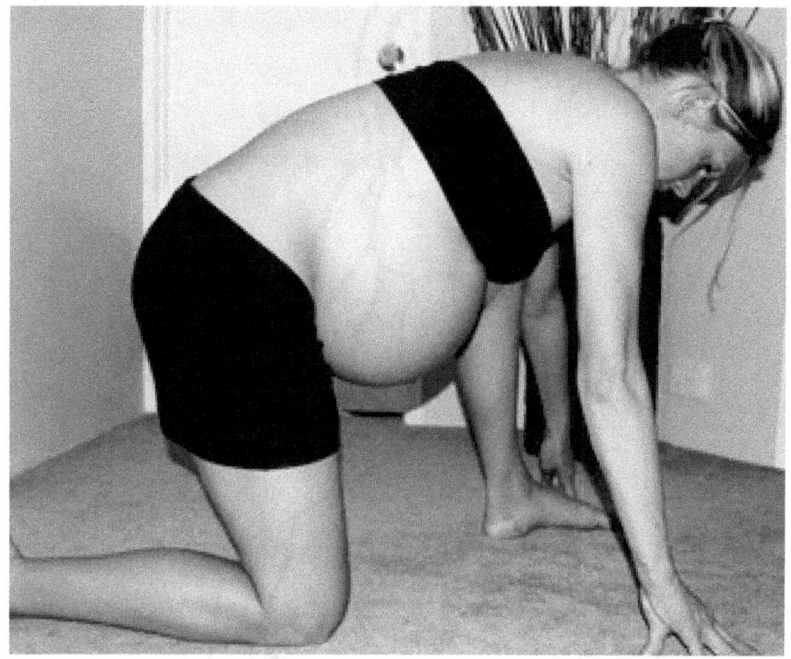

Leaning forward opening the pelvis as seen below

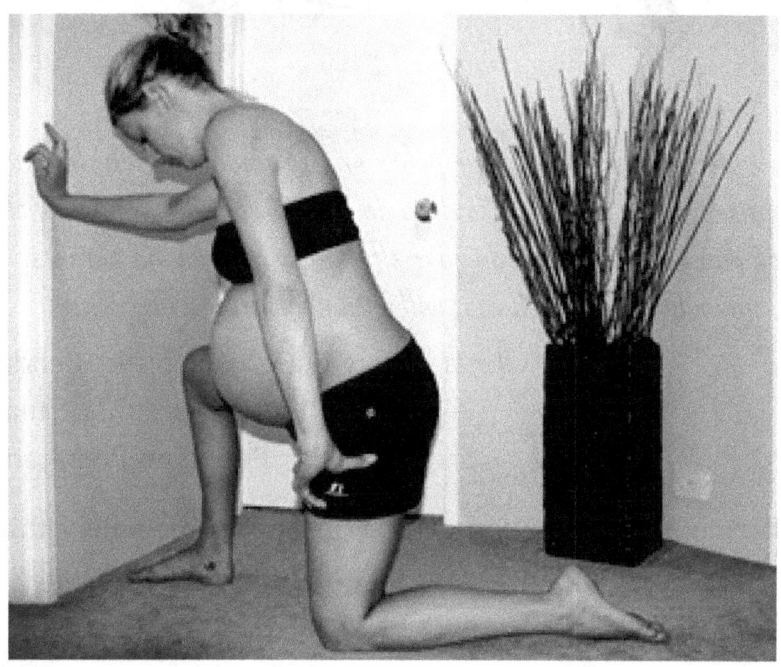

Optimal Foetal Positioning Makes A Labour of Difference!

Sitting on a fitball doing 'ball time' can open up your pelvis.

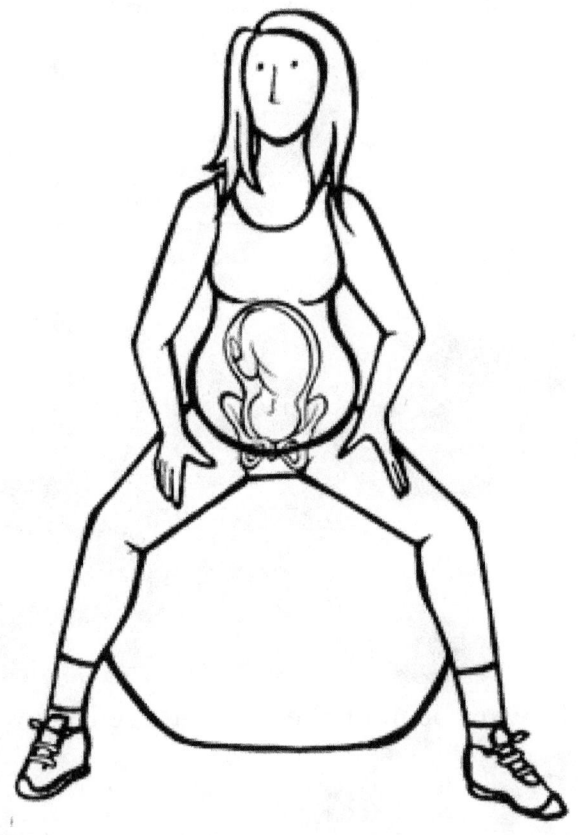

The wider you can open your pelvis and release your tight ligaments the easier it is for you baby to drop down and descend into your pelvis. If you don't have a fitball do yourself a favor and go and purchase one you will not regret it as it will become your new best friend!

Gloria Lemay is a private birth attendant
in Vancouver, B.C., Canada

Perineum Preparation

Perineum preparation can begin at approximately thirty five weeks of pregnancy. This can be done either manually by yourself or your partner or by using an EPI-NO. An EPI-NO is fast becoming very popular for women wanting to have a natural birth experience. The EPI- NO is like a thick rubber balloon which you insert into your vagina, and you pump it up so that it opens this soft tissue gently stretching it. The idea is that you practice using it every couple of days working towards getting the balloon to ten centimetres in dilation. This of course represents the diameter of a baby's head circumference.

I have attended many births where women have been using the EPI-NO and it really does work. I have seen the perineum open so wide and stretch without the need for an episiotomy or a natural tear at all. Even grazes are kept at bay.

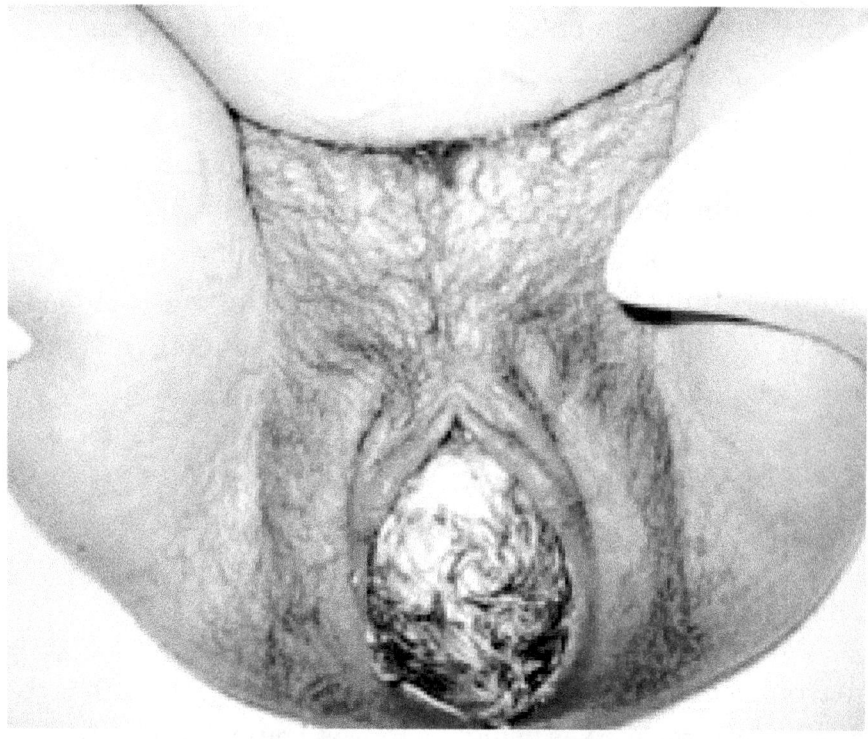

As for manual stretching, this can be done by you or your partner every couple of days. I do recommend that you use my perineum preparation balm which I sell online through my website individually or as part of a labour kit, or a natural cold-pressed oil like apricot, olive or grapeseed. What you will need to do is rub the oil or balm into the perineum before the stretching begins, which will assist in the prevention of tearing and minimise damage by helping this skin tissue to stretch and remain soft and supple throughout the last weeks of pregnancy, leading up to the birth.

" I have seen the perineum open so wide and stretch without the need for an episiotomy or a natural tear at all."

If you are stretching the perineum yourself, the best position to be in is standing up. Put one foot up on a chair, take your arm around behind your bottom and insert two to three fingers into the back of your vagina and pull back on this tissue towards your anus holding for the count of six to eight seconds. You should feel a small amount of discomfort in this area, if you do not it is not stretching the skin! Let go and have a little break, then try it again holding again for six to eight seconds. Perform this at least four to six times per session, pulling a little harder each time so that you can feel yourself stretching a little bit more each time. After a couple of weeks you should feel the difference.

" If it feels nice and you are enjoying it— it is foreplay not peri prep time! There has to be some type of stretchy/intensity or you are not doing it correctly!"

I recently met a Sexologist who told me how she suggests to women to use their sex toys to stretch this tissue which is basically the same idea as using the EPI-NO but with the batteries included! If your partner is going to do your stretching for you, you will need to lie in a slightly reclined position on an armchair or on your bed. Keep your knees bent and your legs opened and relaxed. Your partner will need to place both thumbs into the vagina with oil or balm on them and proceed to push down towards your bottom, holding for about six to eight seconds and then moving his thumbs down and outwards for six to eight seconds as you practice your breathing. He will need to repeat this four to six times over, applying more pressure each and every time. Yes, it will be uncomfortable, and sting a little, so you will need to breathe and focus on letting go. It is great exercise to do in preparation for labour.

Just note: If it feels nice and you are enjoying it—it is foreplay not peri prep time! There has to be some type of stretchy/intensity, or you are not doing it correctly!

9

The Power of Pregnancy And Labour Hormones

As an introduction to this chapter I would like to quote from *Ina May's Guide to Childbirth*, in which she describes her awe and respect for the efficiency and beautiful design of the female body as expressed in labour and birth:

An intricate and exquisitely balanced combination of hormones is necessary to trigger all the right functions of labour and birth. The subtle, complex interplay of exchanging hormone levels during the birth process is one of the most fascinating and little understood aspects of pregnancy and birth in the modern world. Prostaglandins, oxytocin, adrenalin and endorphins are some of the most important natural chemical combinations produced within the woman's body during labour and birth.

The hormones present in the pregnant body during labour play a huge and totally underestimated role. I believe that not enough information about these hormones is provided to women embarking on a natural birth experience. The more information women can be given to gain an understanding of the importance of these hormones, the greater the acknowledgement and acceptance of the wonderful natural process of birth. It is then that a woman in labour can truly tune into her body and be fully aware of exactly what is going on for her in that moment.

Dr Sarah Buckley, Australian mother of four, writes in her paper 'Ecstatic Birth: Natures Hormonal Blueprint for Labour':

Giving birth in ecstasy: This is our birthright and our body's intent. Mother Nature, in her wisdom, prescribes birthing hormones that take us outside ('ec') our usual state ('stasis'), so that we can be transformed on every level as we enter motherhood. This exquisite hormonal orchestration unfolds optimally when birth is undisturbed, enhancing safety for both mother and baby.

When women truly have an insight into the unique interplay of hormones, they can have a far better understanding during labour and birth as to why they are feeling a certain way. Some women do experience a feeling of being 'high' and not on this planet, while other women may feel very calm and relaxed. Others feel uptight and emotional, while some women just feel very primal, like an animal. Whatever the feeling, it is the hormones that are directing, through interplay, the emotions that are present while women are in labour.

When the positive hormones such as endorphins are present in large amounts they truly help a woman to feel comfortable about her body during birth. On the other hand, if catecholamines are present it could be that a woman is feeling anxious and uptight about going into labour. It is important to acknowledge the role of hormones if a woman wants to birth naturally. For example, it is possible to shift a woman in labour out of a negatively controlled hormonal state into a more positive, accepting, surrendering one if she is willing to do so.

Adrenalin And Nonadrenalin – The First Of The Hormones

Adrenalin and nonadrenalin are collectively known as catecholamines. Catecholamines are the fight or flight hormones which are secreted when a person is frightened, fearful or in a potentially dangerous situation. The body releases these hormones in response to external stress.

These hormones are produced in the brain, the adrenal glands on top of the kidneys and in the nerve endings around the body. They act on the nerve endings of the sympathetic nervous system and produce what is known as the 'fight or flight' response.

When a woman goes into labour and she is hesitant, reluctant and fearful, she will often be producing catecholamines, which will further cause her to stay in a frightened, scared frame of mind. She may experience the need to have pain relief as she may be fighting the need to just surrender and go with the flow of contractions.

Catecholamine production during labour can result in:

- Failure to progress – because a woman may be fighting the contractions instead of working with them.
- Not going into established labour – labour starts off very slowly but does not get into a substantial rhythm; the woman may be feeling anxious and restless and not mentally or physically prepared to let go and surrender, therefore pro- ducing catecholamines, which further inhibit the labour.
- Poorly coordinated uterine action – the contractions of the

uterus may not be strong enough or rhythmical enough to start the dilation of the cervix.

Some of the possible signs a woman is not ready to surrender and go into early labour are due to catecholamines being released as a result of anxiety and panic behaviour. (Please note that these refer to early labour signs only). She may show signs of:

- being restless/agitated.
- the need to make loud noises.
- moving wildly in an annoyed manner.
- constant activity.
- wide, staring eyes.
- raised blood pressure.
- increased and excessive pain on contractions.
- all of the above, due to extreme fear and anxiety about allowing oneself to let go and surrender to the contractions as they find their own natural rhythm.

Ways to avoid and slow down the production of catecholamines

- Identify the source of fear or disturbance and remove it, talk about it – verbally express what it is that you fear.
- Provide privacy in a small, safe environment: e.g. the toilet, bath or a quiet familiar room will often calm a woman down, making her feel safe.
- Avoid unnecessary procedures, e.g. regular internal examinations.
- Change the environment, e.g. dim the lights, play some calming music, get into the shower or bath.
- Reduce the number of people and activities in the room.

- Provide continuity of care from the support person/s – if supporting, don't leave the room!
- Allow time for adrenalin to decrease and the endorphins to override – at least one hour in a new environment.
- Support persons should whisper to the woman in labour and avoid eye contact or full conversations (unless they instigate it) and try not to question them about things.
- Try counselling and offering positive affirmations, e.g. by telling this person their body is doing a wonderful job, that their body is designed to birth a baby, etc.

Protecting The Neocortex Of The Brain

As Ina May Gaskin, a delightful American author (*Spiritual Midwifery* and *Ina May's Guide to Childbirth*), suggests, it is important that women keep out of the neocortex of their brain. It is the neocortex that is responsible for the thought processes evoked when a woman is asked a question. Being exposed to bright lights when in labour can have the same effect, as can failing to protect her privacy. A woman's best chance of staying in a safe labour state is to assist her to stay in the primitive part of her brain, which has the primary role of keeping her in an inner place, where it is safe to open up and give birth. As a care provider and support person this is your primary role.

Adrenalin In The Baby

The baby also produces catecholamines, but this is a positive rather than a negative response to labour. As the uterus contracts there is reduced blood flow to the placenta. However, to counteract this problem the placenta stores oxygenated blood between contractions, to ensure that when a contraction takes place the baby has adequate amounts of oxygen. The baby can also internally shunt blood through its body to its brain, heart and lungs to prevent hypoxia (lack of oxygen). Adrenalin immobilises energy stores in the baby's body, which helps it to survive during these times of reduced oxygen availability.

Endorphins – the natural helper during labour and a woman's best assistant!

Endorphins are neuropeptides – natural opiates which the body produces in the pituitary gland to make us feel calm and relaxed. Their effect is ten times greater than that of morphine and is similar to that of pethidine and heroin which, coincidentally, work on the same receptors of the brain. Endorphins are produced in the brain stem, nerve endings and the placenta.

In *Birthing from Within*, Pam England and Rob Horowitz state:

When the brain perceives pain (especially with the added stimulus of stress) endorphins are released. Endorphins are chemical compounds secreted by the brain and adrenal glands and have a pain-relieving effect ten times more potent than morphine.

As dilation progresses the sensation of pain will increase. The more pain you have, the more endorphins are released to help you cope. The rising level of endorphins contributes to a shift from a thinking, rational mindset to a more primitive and instinctive one. Hence, it really is a good idea during labour to try to keep 'out of your head' and not to analyse why this or that is happening. Instead, just let your body do what is necessary and put the thinking, logical part of your brain on hold temporarily. Endorphins take you to a dreamlike state, which meshes well with the tasks of birthing. Endorphins are also mood elevators, for example by producing 'a runner's high'.

The main effect endorphins have during labour:

- They modify the pain – the intensity of pain may feel less than it actually is.
- They create a sense of wellbeing – women may feel very calm and blissful.
- They alter the sense of time – women often totally lose track of time.
- They make women forget about the pain after the baby is born – like amnesia, women almost always forget about the intensity of the labour immediately after the birth.

Endorphin production is at its highest point during the transition phase of labour, which explains why a lot of women find it hard to remember the pain associated with the pushing part of the birth. At the height of the pushing stage the endorphin production helps a woman to manage the pain and assists her to focus inwardly to work her baby out of her body.

The endorphins can make a woman in labour look very relaxed, as if she is on drugs, seeming drunk or stoned. Her motions and the way she perceives things around her change. More often than not, a woman needs lots of time to process information and respond when being asked a question. Too much information or too many questions can cause a woman to start producing adrenalin, in response to feeling overwhelmed and out of control.

Endorphins are the friendly guys to have on board during labour. Therefore it is imperative that support people and care providers assist a woman in staying calm, comfortable, relaxed and honoured in the choices she makes. This allows labour to flow very easily and aids the outcome of a natural vaginal birth.

Oxytocin – The *Feel Good* Hormone

Oxytocin is one of the hormones responsible for contractions of the uterus throughout a woman's life, during menstruation, pregnancy, labour and birth. The milk ejection reflex is also initiated by oxytocin. During labour, oxytocin is considered the accelerator of birth as it speeds up labour by stimulating the contractions to be strong and dynamic. Oxytocin is made and released from the hypothalamus in our brain and then stored in the posterior pituitary gland. It is released in response to stimulation of certain sites, integral to reproduction behaviours. Oxytocin helps to:

- create smooth rhythmical contractions of the uterine muscles.
- make contractions feel like an orgasmic experience for some women.
- condition a woman to want to have her baby in a biological way, consolidating her need to have a strong bonding process.
- assist the cervix to totally open up as the baby descends to allow the baby's head to pass through.
- prevent postpartum haemorrhage due to high levels of oxytocin being present when mother and baby have skin-to-skin contact immediately after birth.
- create a breast milk 'ejection' or 'let down reflex' so breast milk will start to flow when a woman feels her baby near the breast or hears her baby cry.

Factors which inhibit oxytocin production:

- fear and anxiety
- external factors – transferring to hospital from home during labour, unknown people being present, bright lights, distractions, feeling exposed
- internal fears – being worried about the baby, fear of the pain, fear of perineal tearing
- interventions such as induction and augmentation (synthetic oxytocin – Syntocinon or Pitocin – from an external source), which flood the receptor sites with abnormally high levels of oxytocin and render the body less sensitive to levels needed, so the brain reduces the natural production during labour
- an epidural – this interferes with and numbs the receptor sites involved in the initiation and production of oxytocin
- episiotomy – this reduces the stretch of the perineum, hence there is no oxytocin release as receptor-site feedback is reduced, which could lead to severe postpartum haemorrhage

Prostaglandins

The prostaglandins are produced by the uterus during pregnancy and are known to increase during spontaneous term labour. The prostaglandins are said to stimulate uterine muscle activity, which triggers an increase in oxytocin levels, required to initiate labour. Natural prostaglandins start the process of thinning out the cervix and ripening the birth-canal tissue in preparation for childbirth.

It is interesting that male sperm is also a form of natural prostaglandins, hence having a male ejaculate into the vagina/cervix can stimulate the cervix tissue enough to instigate contractions and tightening of the uterine muscles. This is a wonderful way to get things going if a woman is 'overdue', and the pressure is on, from the medical care providers, for a woman to go into labour. It doesn't work for everybody but you can have fun trying!

When a woman is induced through artificial means a synthetic prostaglandin E2 suppository is inserted into the vagina. The difference between the real thing, sperm, and the manmade suppository, is that the latter is about twenty times stronger, causing a quicker reaction from the cervix. This method does not take into account the woman's own internal contraction of her muscles during orgasm when she is having sex, with her partner ejaculating at the same time. However, with either scenario the onset of labour will still only occur if a woman is ready. Nothing in the way of drugs, synthetic or the real deal, will budge a closed, un-ripened cervix. This is why patience is a virtue that needs to be learned by tired, heavy pregnant women!

The foetus ejection reflex

This is a rather ugly medical term for an incredible aspect of a woman's body! The following is an extract from *Ina May's Guide to Childbirth*, which dramatically illustrates this reflex:

My sister's first birth was an example of adrenalin having the opposite effect – of speeding up labour instead of slowing it down. When an impatient doctor warned her that a cesarean would be necessary if she wasn't fully dilated in twenty minutes, she managed to dilate the five centimeters necessary to escape surgery. 'I really didn't want to get cut!'

she later told me. French physician Michel Odent calls my sister's experience an example of the fetal ejection reflex – a sudden rise in adrenalin gives us the surge of power necessary to complete the job and birth.

When a woman is in very established labour and is suddenly faced with a fearful situation, for example the idea of a forceps delivery or having a C-section, this may be enough of a stimulant to cause a huge production of adrenalin. This huge surge causes the cervix to dilate completely and powerful contractions occur that cause the baby to be expelled from the body very quickly. This is known as the foetal ejection reflex.

During normal transition, adrenalin production is needed to get a baby out of the body. Women can slowly dilate to maximum cervical stretch, but one thing that is present in either slow or fast birthing scenarios is the type of verbal comment made by a woman, such as:

> *'Just get the baby out.' 'I want to die.'*
> *'Leave me alone.' 'Don't touch me.'*
> *'I can't take any more of this.' 'When is it going to end?'*
> *'Just give me a C-section.'*

This type of spoken dialogue is normal and directly related to transition and the release of adrenalin within the body. Another direct result of adrenalin being produced at transition is that fully dilated women may also vomit.

Relaxin – a pregnancy hormone and a woman's best friend

The hormone relaxin is produced throughout pregnancy, from as early as four weeks after conception. The further a woman progresses, the greater the production of relaxin. By the time a woman is due the relaxin present in her body provides her with great extensibility and pliability of ligaments and muscles, so the pelvic bones can open and move, allowing the baby to pass through.

While the pelvis may feel like a stiff, ridged group of bones it can actually pull apart with the assistance of relaxin in loosening the ligaments that hold it together. If these bones did not open and shift during labour it would be difficult to birth a baby through the pelvis. Nature has been very kind in providing the adequate tools to allow this to occur naturally. So there is a reason why women weren't provided with a zip above the pubic area after all!

This wonderful hormone is also responsible for the movement of other joints. Movement of the sacroiliac joint can cause problems for a pregnant woman. Opening and shifting of the pelvic bones in late pregnancy can give the sensation that the baby is going to fall out of the body. Sometimes a woman can feel so open through the pelvic area that if she sits on the toilet and pushes it seems that the baby may just fall out! This sensation is very much the result of the relaxin hormone kicking in, making everything feel stretched and open, ready for the baby's journey to the outside world.

The relaxin hormone can also make women look very soft in their face; I call it the hormonal look. Sometimes when you talk to a pregnant woman they can appear very vague and away with the fairies – *like the lights are on but no one is home!* (I mean that in the nicest possible way!) Pregnancy can be very calm and peaceful, a time of focus within, in preparation for birth. It is hard to fight the vagueness, and women who are still at work regularly com- ment to me that very little work is being done as it becomes so hard to concentrate – instead they find themselves daydreaming and losing their train of thought.

The relaxin hormone can make women very forgetful. I lost my purse full of money after shopping one day, only to find it in the fridge later on that night. A woman who came to my class told me how she got onto the wrong bus in Perth and ended up down south, nearly an hour from the city, before she finally realised. The relaxin hormone does just that: it relaxes not only the body, but the mind as well, to such a degree that we can often forget what our purpose actually is in doing something or going somewhere.

And finally – the uncontrollable collective of hormones that cause the nesting instinct or the need to renovate!

Many women have turned up to my classes at the pool totally exhausted because they have been cleaning obsessively all day. I tell them it's because they are nesting.

Some women just can't stop, they clean from sun-up to sundown, while others tell me they have bursts of nesting for a couple of hours a day. The unusual thing about nesting is that often these women will clean parts of their house that they would never normally touch. I often ask, 'Have you cleaned the oven yet?' If they reply that they have, I know they have the nesting bug pretty bad. Who ever really wants to clean their oven? I can remember being obsessed about the oven being clean during every pregnancy – this was my nesting bugbear.

Nesting is totally natural and normal and nearly all women nest in some way during the course of their pregnancy. What nesting is really about is creating and establishing an environment that a woman feels is ideal to bring a baby into. For some reason, by having a clean oven, or clean fridge, or clean hand-scrubbed floor, the baby is going to be better off!

Nesting may also be seen in cooking. Women will tell me that they have been baking all day. I ask, 'What were you baking?' They reply, 'All sorts of things, from cakes to home-made pizzas to apple pie.' Other women start to knit or sew baby clothes, such as beanies and booties or complete outfits.

The other very common thing that tends to run through my antenatal classes is the amount of renovating that goes on in the home prior to a baby being born. The idea, of course, is that a woman and her partner want to have the house looking as great as possible so the baby feels comfortable and secure. I have to mention that the baby is not really going to notice the difference between the old and the new, so don't bust yourself too much as it could turn out to be to your body's or baby's detriment if you overdo it.

There is another major 'nesting' process that grabs some people – the urge to put their home on the market just prior to a baby arriving. More often than not a couple will not have found a new place to buy or rent, as they can't decide on what they want to do. As scary as this predicament seems, lots of couples, and more so the woman, appear totally relaxed and calm about the whole thing. This is probably due to the relaxin hormone kicking in. They will often state,

The reason women are so affected by the hormones in pregnancy is to slow them down and get them to focus within, shutting out the world and all the unnecessary noise and distractions of life.

'I'm not worried as I just feel so calm and relaxed that everything will work out in the end.' Of course, it always does, and the baby is oblivious to everything, including the colour of the paint on the walls and the newly polished floorboards!

10

Avoiding The Fear-Tension-Pain Syndrome

It is an honour to present the fear–tension–pain theory that Dr Grantly Dick-Read discovered in the early twentieth century. He was one of the earliest known obstetricians to gain the understanding that women can birth without fear and in a relaxed, calm manner if they are given the opportunity and courage to do so.

I have taken the following quotes from his book *Childbirth Without Fear*, first published in 1942. He is the man who began the job of changing the way that women saw childbirth at that time (and still do to this present day). The work of Grantly Dick-Read is also the premise on which a lot of today's natural childbirth educational books are written.

Dick-Read was a great scientist, philosopher and medical practitioner who demonstrated an understanding of the natural ability of the body to birth way before any of his counterparts. His observations of women wanting to experience natural childbirth started when he came across a woman labouring in a dark, cold room. When asked by Dr Dick-Read if she wanted to be given chloroform, she refused.

Chloroform is a drug poured into a mask and placed over the face of a woman to knock her out during labour. Back in those times, it was common practice for a woman to be knocked out cold and have the baby pulled from her body with forceps! The idea was that no woman should have to suffer the 'extreme' amount of pain that accompanies childbirth. The pain of childbirth was incomprehensible to the doctors of that time, and it is frequently seen in the same light today – being viewed as 'too much' for a woman to bear a child naturally.

When the woman was asked afterwards why she had refused the mask for chloroform, she paused and did not reply for some time, then said, *'It didn't hurt. It wasn't meant to, was it, Doctor?'*

This observation started his exploration into why some women have absolutely no pain associated with childbirth. He began questioning the possibility that childbirth pain had an association with how a woman perceives her labour contractions. He also began to question that if a woman does not perceive labour contractions to be painful, more often than not they will *not be painful*. Gradually his understanding of the relationships between the mind, fear and pain led to the development of his fear–tension–pain theory.

Dick-Read noted that when women were not watched over or observed by someone and when they were free from fear they actually birthed with considerable ease and little to no pain. The muscles of the cervix relaxed and opened and they could push their baby out themselves with very little resistance.

Dick-Read gained a better understanding of the concept of fear–tension–pain through further observation of labouring women, a concept that took another seventy years to explain scientifically! Who would have thought that the body would have a built-in natural analgesia that helps women to stay calm and relaxed when in labour. The body opiates known as 'endorphins' are the body's natural painkillers. Studies by scientists have shown that the opiate molecules lock on to special receptor sites of neurons in the central nervous system, slowing down the firing rate of these neurons, hence slowing down the rate at which we experience childbirth sensations.

This is why women find that having massage and hands on pressure on the lower back, or hot water and pressure from the shower head, a hot pack on the lower back, or being completely submersed in a bath of hot steamy water is so wonderful – it decreases the intensity being felt, registered by the pain receptors located in and around the pelvis, spine and lower back.

It is important to note here that many of the neuron sites are located in the spinal cord, where pain sensations are processed by the body.

Slowing down the firing rate of neurons results in a decreased sense of pain and suppresses the synaptic activity of the brain, producing a tranquil, calm, amnesiac state. This is what I call the 'labour look', which is when a woman looks hormonal and soft in her eyes, becomes slow in her talking and thinking and needs time to respond to questions. Her brain is basically slowing down and moving into this lovely birth state. This actually assists a woman to remain calm and mellow, totally surrendering to the internal sensations of her body.

The fear–tension–pain theory is based on Dr Dick-Read's understanding that if a woman *fears* the birth of her baby, her body is going to respond by becoming *tense* (the muscles don't contract well), which will lead to a more exacerbated *pain* sensation during contractions. This can become a continuous cycle if a woman is not aware of it, and eventually it results in labour not progressing or a woman not experiencing regular contractions at all. Worse, a woman may feel so overwhelmed by every contraction that she becomes terrified and scared as the next contraction begins.

Sometimes fear-based issues can be just under the surface and do not come out until a woman goes into labour, in which case a woman will have to deal with whatever arises. However, more often than not, women can identify relatively early in their pregnancy what they have fears about.

A good way to identify fears around childbirth and mothering is to talk in a group with other pregnant women. Women may have to form their own group or seek out an independent childbirth class where there is an opportunity to express yourself freely and openly and be heard. The thing to look for in a group is that it is supportive of your particular needs and non-judgemental, so that you can allow your fears to surface, be spoken about and addressed through open discussion.

To prevent the Fear-Tension-Pain cycle from being an issue during labour, it is important for a pregnant woman to assess and evaluate what she is fearing about labour and giving birth, then seek help to release this prior to giving birth, so she can avoid this cycle.

The more open, clear-minded and positive women can be as their baby's estimated arrival time approaches, the easier it is to go into labour free from fear–tension–pain. It is possible for women to experience a positive birth in any setting, whether it be in the hospital or at home, if the appropriate mental preparation has been done. Mental preparation, especially identifying fears, must be of the utmost importance to a pregnant woman. Saying, 'I'll just see what happens on the day' will just not cut it, I'm afraid. If our thoughts really do create our reality, then we have to put lots of time and energy into acknowledging what we are programming into our thoughts and belief systems.

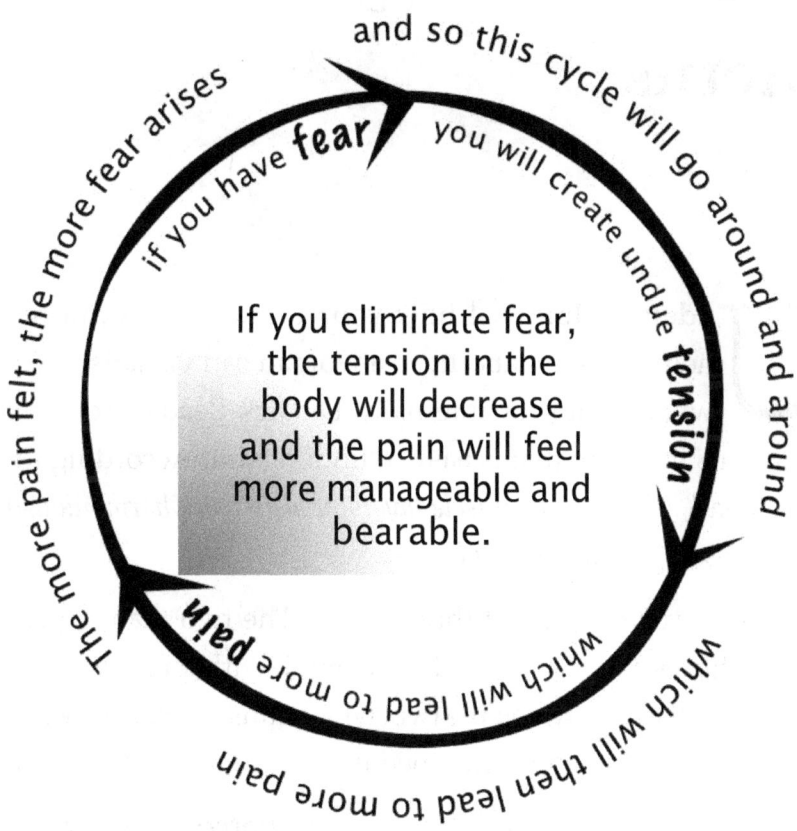

A representation of the cyclic pathway to show in more modern terms the concept of Dr Grantly Dick-Read's fear–tension–pain theory.

11

Understanding Your Uterus

Understanding just how your uterus works can really help when in labour, so a woman can visualise exactly what is going on internally. Dr Dick-Read has described the uterus in a way that is easy to understand. According to Dr Dick-Read, *'the uterine muscle layers need to work harmoniously if birthing is to go smoothly and easily.'*

The uterus consists of three layers. The two main layers of muscle fibres are vertical and horizontal, with an inner layer of connective tissue between the two, which runs in many directions, matted closely together, entwined in a figure-of-eight formation.

The inner layer of muscle fibres is the horizontal one and the fibres are closely bunched together in the lower part of the uterus. The main function of these muscles is to contract and tighten in a wave-like action to push and squeeze the baby downwards until the cervix is fully open.

The outer layer of vertical muscle fibres is responsible for contracting and shortening the uterus and pulling the cervix outwards and upwards, allowing the baby to pass through the neck of the uterus and into the birth canal.

When the two sets of muscles are simultaneously working in harmony, the uterus will open naturally and function appropriately, and the baby will move downwards into the birth canal to be born.

The following diagram has been included to assist you to gain a visual understanding of the three sets of muscles more clearly.

The Laws Of The Sphincter

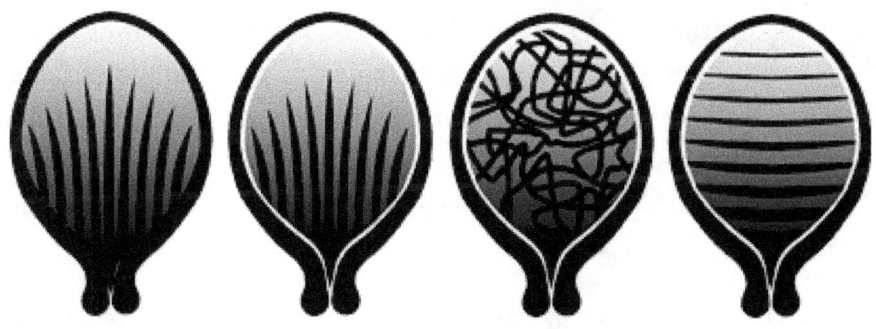

I have to say that I have never in my wildest thoughts considered the birth canal and vagina as a sphincter of the body! So it is with great pleasure that I present the teachings of Ina May Gaskin, whom I met some years ago at a homebirth conference in Western Australia. Ina May explains that:

Sphincters are circular muscle groups that ordinarily remain contracted so the openings of certain organs are held closed until something needs to pass through. Each sphincter's job is to relax and expand so that it can open comfortably and wide enough to allow the passage of what ever must move through. Elimination and birthing both involve the opening of the sphincters.

The laws of the sphincter, according to Ina May, are:

- Excretory, cervical and vaginal sphincters function best in an atmosphere of intimacy and privacy – for example, a bathroom with a locking door, or a bedroom, where interruption is unlikely or impossible.

- These sphincters cannot be opened at will and do not respond well to commands (such as 'Push!' or 'Relax!').

- When a person's sphincter is in the process of opening, it may suddenly close down if that person becomes upset, frightened, humiliated, or self-conscious. Why? High levels of adrenalin in the bloodstream do not favour (sometimes they actually prevent) the opening of the sphincters. This inhibition factor is one important reason why women in tra- ditional societies have mostly chosen other women – except in extraordinary circumstances – to attend them in labour and birth.

- The state of relaxation of the mouth and jaw is directly correlated to the ability of the cervix, the vagina and the anus to open to full capacity. An open mouth and relaxed jaw can help the vagina and cervix to open. (I suggest you remember this if you ever suffer from haemorrhoids and are afraid to poop, as this aspect of the Sphincter Law is helpful in that situation as well as during birthing.)

Another interesting point to note about sphincters is they often respond well to laughter. This is a positive way to help the sphincters relax and release – in fact, laughter can be an effective form of anaesthesia.

Deep abdominal breathing can also assist the body and allow general all-over relaxation, including the pelvic-floor muscles. Being immersed in a big tub of hot water also enables deep relaxation, hence supporting the opening of the sphincters.

Another interesting point of Ina May's is that sphincters can suddenly close when their owner is startled or frightened. The sudden contraction of previously relaxed sphincter muscles is a fear-based reaction. This is part of the natural fight-or-flight response to perceived danger. Adrenalin and catecholamines rise in the bloodstream when a person is frightened or angered. Female animals in labour in the wild, such as gazelles and wildebeest, can be on the point of giving birth and yet suddenly reverse the process if surprised by a predator! This is just one of the ways that all mammals have programmed-in protection during the vulnerable process of labour and birth.

These same evolutionary behaviours exist in humans when we go into labour, without us necessarily understanding the evolutionary wisdom of our own reactions. Hence, it is very important to feel as comfortable as possible in one's surroundings and to eliminate any stress and anxiety before and during labour. Creating an environment conducive to natural birthing is of utmost importance and should be given great thought and preparation prior to labour, in order to assist your sphincters to open and stay open.

12

Changing The Birthing Room To Suit Your Needs And Progress Your Labour

Not everyone decides on a homebirth. If you are headed for hospital, then the best way to stay in deep labour once you have entered a hospital labour room is to change the setting immediately to suit your needs and to make you feel as comfortable as possible.

Ask the hospital staff or get your support person/persons to find, bring, arrange or set up in your room the following:

- mattress for the floor
- fitball to sit on
- beanbag to rest on/over
- bluetooth speaker so you can put on calming music
- an electric oil-burner to make the room smell beautiful and to get rid of the hospital smell (note – you cannot usually have an open-flame burner or candles in the hospital)

- lights to be dimmed so it is not so bright in the room
- your favorite doona, blanket or sheets near you
- your birth plan hung on the walls, for all to see and read
- positive birthing affirmations for you and your support people to read

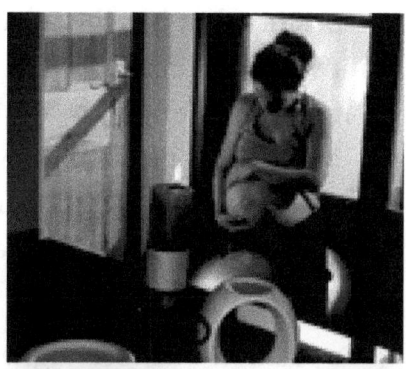
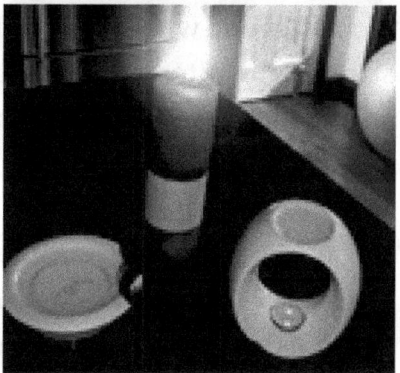
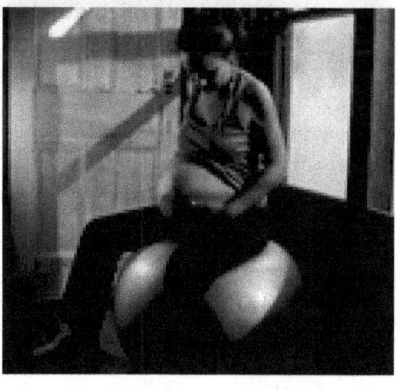

All of the above will do wonders for a stark, white-walled room where the emphasis is usually on the bed, which is often situated in the middle of the room. Push the bed up against the wall so you have more space to move (and so there is less opportunity to get up on the bed and onto your back). Staying comfortable off the bed and remaining 'passively active', moving about in a space that you feel relaxed in, can assist you to keep labouring for a great length of time.

Staying 'Passively Active' During Labour

What exactly is being 'passively active'? This is a term that I use to describe a woman in labour who is basically staying in one position but has the freedom to move about on the spot in that position or change to another position. It is a balance between being active and passive. It is having the freedom to move on the spot or to travel.

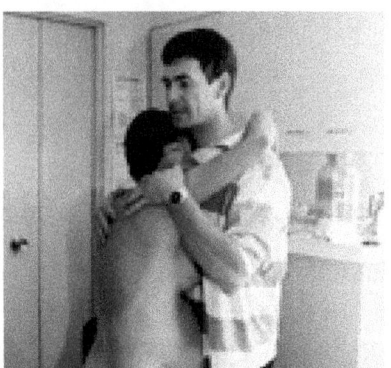

A position that feels right to a woman is one where she can have strong and intense contractions and not feel like she has to move. I am yet to meet a woman who tells me she is happy on her back or on her side while in labour! These positions should not be suggested, as they can be incredibly uncomfortable when a contraction comes on.

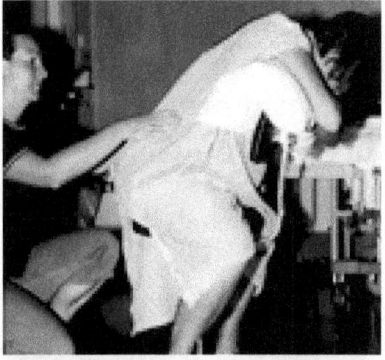

Some of the positions below are suitable to suggest to a labouring woman, if you are a support person. However, it is always the woman's choice as to what position she wants to be in, what she wants to stay with or try out. Women in labour can be encouraged to try out as many options as possible till they find what suits them best at the time. This, of course, may change from hour to hour as they experience the different stages of labour.

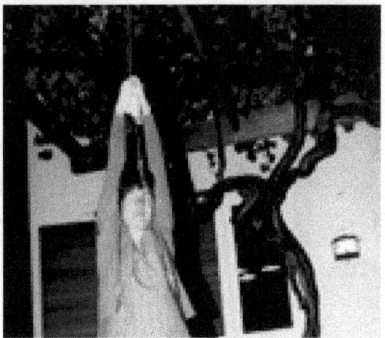

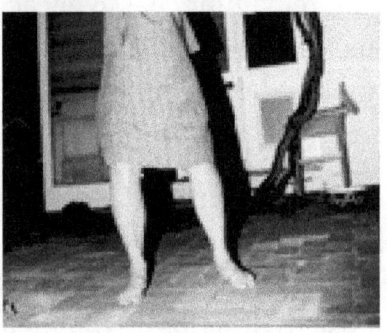

Below are some options:

- Standing up – leaning over against the wall, hanging off partner's neck/shoulders, or bending over a high change-table, the back of a chair or bench.

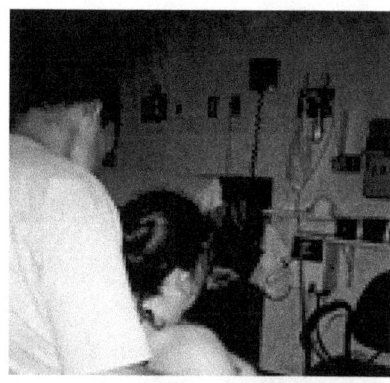

- Sitting on a fitball – a woman can bounce, rock, sway or rotate her body and pelvis. Leaning over a bed while on the fitball can be a very comfortable position.

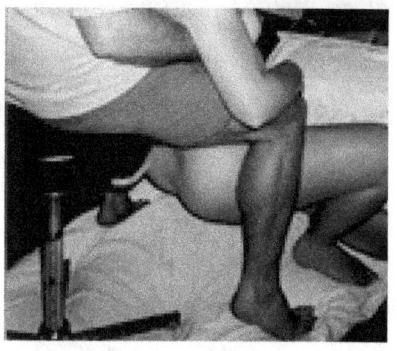

- Hanging off a rope or bar during contractions can be wonderful as gravity really goes to work!

- Getting on all fours, hands and knees on the floor, bed or on a foam mattress on the floor can really help if the labour pain is all in the back due to a posterior positioning of the baby (baby's spine to mother's spine).

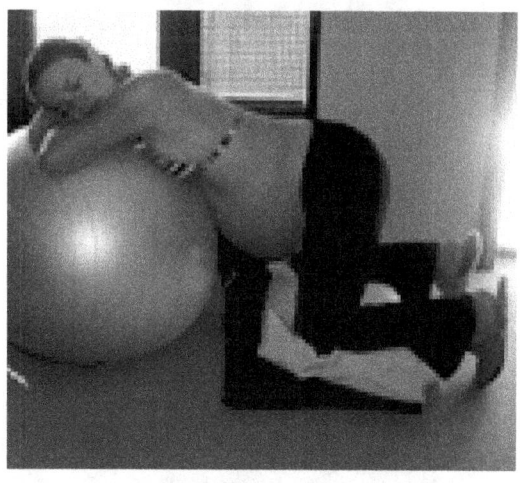

- Kneeling forward works really well when in a birthing tub, or putting your head onto a pillow on a chair, bed, beanbag, or your partner's lap.

- Squatting – holding on to a chair, partner or bed for support really enables the pelvis to open up incredibly.
- Floating in a big tub of hot water and stretching out in a horizontal position can be wonderful and very relaxing as no weight is placed on the body in water. Pam England writes:

Laying on your back during labour literally collapses the pelvis, distorting its natural opening, and decreasing its natural diameter by as much as an inch! Squatting, on the other hand, relaxes the pubic symphysis and increases the pubic arch, the space under the pubic bones, which is necessary to rotate the head in the birth canal. The sacroiliac joint also gives the sacrum flexibility.

When the trunk bends forward, as it does in the squatting position, the sacrum turns on its axis and opens up the pelvis from behind, increasing the width of the pelvic outlet by twenty-five per cent.

It really does make sense to stay off the bed for the very reason that we lose the benefit of gravity to assist us in birth. Lying on a bed forces women to push uphill. I feel that at the pushing stage of labour women need all the help they can get from gravity, and, as Pam England suggests, the twenty-five per cent in extra space makes a really big difference to the birth outlet.

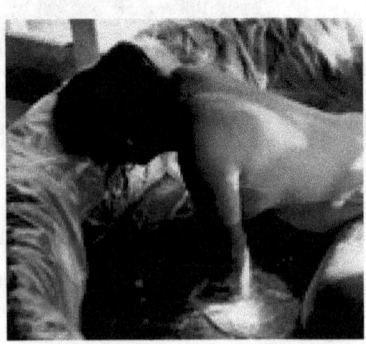 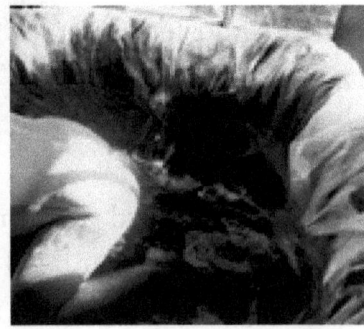

13

What Are The Benefits of Having A Natural Childbirth?

Natural childbirth means no physical, chemical or psychological condition likely to disturb the normal sequence of events or disrupt the natural phenomenon of parturition. Grantly Dick-Read.

I believe that by learning about natural childbirth women can gain a clear understanding about why it is so important that the body be given the opportunity to 'do the job it is designed to do'.

Having said that, I also know that sometimes the body does this job incredibly slowly and women burn out. It is just not meant to be, in some birth situations. And for whatever reason, unexpected scenarios can and do arise from time to time and I do acknowledge the importance of medical help when there are true complications.

What is important is that you prepare and plan for the best possible outcome and do not doubt yourself or your body's ability. Expect only the best for you and your baby and you will be setting yourself up for a positive outcome. If you dwell on the 'what if' and the 'I don't know about all of this' you could be programming your mind and body for a very different outcome. Of course, whatever your birthing experience, the end result will be that you have a baby in your arms, but the real challenge is in the journey to bring the baby into this world and exposing yourself and the baby to all the wonderful hormones and possibilities available.

I often ask women if they had a choice to go down road A, which represents a natural childbirth with a quick recovery, or road B, which represents lots of intervention and a slower recovery, which would they choose? The majority always choose to travel down road A. They acknowledge without hesitation that there are far more positives about that journey – the journey of pain, surrender, emotional connection, triumph, pure ecstasy and elation, rather than the experience that road B offers. Road B is often the complete opposite, with no emotional satisfaction derived at all from the experience. In fact, many women feel dis- empowered and angry after a birth full of interventions.

Here are some benefits of having a natural childbirth:

- The body that goes into labour naturally and spontaneously gets a nice 'warm up'. That is, mild contractions that are very manageable slowly building in intensity to stronger, slightly longer contractions over a given time.
- Nature is very kind in that it usually allows plenty of recovery time in between contractions, so women can rest and allow their body and mind to recover before the next contraction.
- When a woman goes into labour naturally she has started

her birth process in a very positive way, which assists her to feel strong and determined. The birthing hormones will be increased due to this mental state, giving a heightened sense of wellbeing that assists a woman to go further into a deep, focused state, enabling her to labour for a great length of time, surrendering with no hesitation or doubts.

- Making the choice not to have drugs during labour helps prevent a cascade of interventions even beginning. The effects of drugs often leads to further interventions, which can ultimately result in needing a Caesarean.
- A woman can be totally aware of all that is going on around her, even while she is in a labour space because she has no internal interference with blood pressure, heart rate or the physical and emotional state of the normal body. This is due to the absence of chemical opiates/drugs being present in the bloodstream interfering with the natural, normal state of the body.
- There will be no interference or crossing over to the placenta of chemical opiates/drugs of any kind that may cause problems for the baby's heart rate, pulse, or sucking reflex after the birth. A baby will come out fully charged on birth hormones, alert and ready to feed.
- Recovery time will be very quick with a short time of vaginal discomfort for most women.
- Mother/baby maternal bonding is increased, as mum is able to lift and cuddle baby with immediate skin-to-skin contact, with minimal problems or discomfort.
- The chances of postnatal depression (PND) are reduced as a woman who has given birth naturally is charged with hormones and often feels invincible and empowered to cope

with any future stresses or problems. Conversely, a birth full of medical interventions, if not handled respectfully, can often lead to a woman feeling disempowered; there has been some preliminary research indicating that women who experience a disempowering birth may have a higher risk of developing PND.

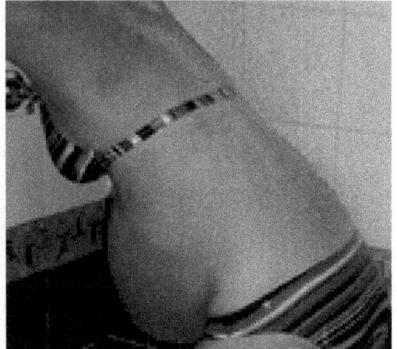

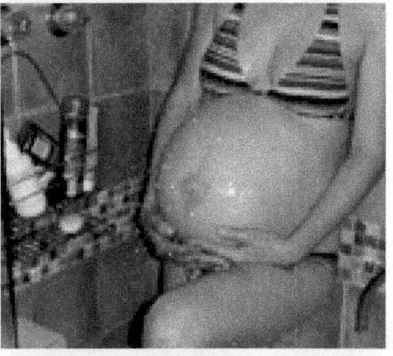

- Natural birth is the most rewarding and amazing experience a woman can go through – it can leave her on a high for days, even weeks.

- A woman can get up off the floor or bed, get out of the birthing tub and walk around, take a shower, or go to the toilet due to having the full sensation and feeling in her body.

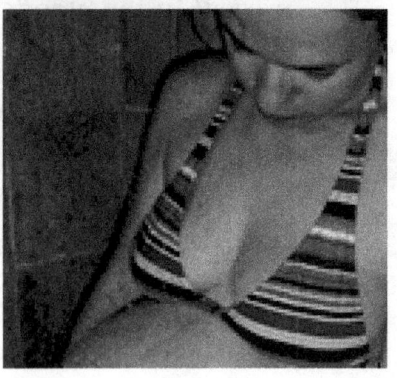

- The postnatal woman experiences a form of amnesia that assists her to completely forget what she has just experienced, that is, the intensity of the contractions, therefore allowing her to totally focus on the baby and breastfeeding.

The interesting thing about pain is that it is clean. When you are finished experiencing pain, it is over. You cannot re-experience its sensation by remembering it. Labour pain is a special type of pain: It almost always happens without causing any damage to the body.
Ina May Gaskin.

14

Natural Pain-Relief Methods

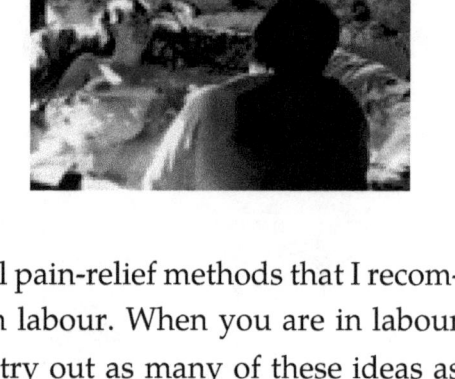

Here is a list of natural pain-relief methods that I recommend for women in labour. When you are in labour it is a good idea to try out as many of these ideas as possible to see what gives you the best relief from the intensity of the contrac- tions. Your support person can remember to suggest different positions, so that you only need to concentrate on managing the contractions.

It's also a good idea to move from one method to the next, as if in a circuit class going from station to station, staying at one station for as long as it feels really comfortable for you. If you feel you really love the hot tub, stay there as long as you can. However, if you feel you need to move or do something different, go with your own intuition and move. This can help pass the time incredibly quickly.

Natural pain-relief methods:

- A big deep bath, spa or warm pool.
- A hot shower.
- Massage on the lower back.
- Hot packs, wheat bags or gel packs for lower back and lower belly.
- TENS (Transcutaneous Electrical Nerve Stimulation) machine (not really natural, but is not a drug and acts as a distracter).
- Hypnosis for Birth: deep, guided relaxation/meditation.
- Breathing in a rhythmical manner: this helps to keep a woman focusing on her breath, which then coincides with her contractions.

The Gate Theory Of Pain Control

The Gate Theory was created in 1970 by Wall and Melzack, to try to offer an explanation as to why women in labour experience pain modification when fully immersed in water compared to just being in gravity. The following is their explanation as cited in Janet Balaskas and Yehudi Gordon's book *Water Birth: The Concise Guide to Water for Pregnancy, Birth and Infancy*:

All sensations converge in the dorsal horn of the spinal cord. Pain sensations are modified or partially 'gated out' by competing sensations of warmth and touch on the mother's skin when she is immersed in water during labour. Hence, this is the reason why women in labour love lower back massage, heat packs and hot water on their back!

The dorsal horn extends the entire length of the spinal cord. Impulses from the nerves all over the body, arising from stimuli such as pain, touch or temperature, converge in the dorsal horn and are transmitted to the brain.

In other words, the nerve endings in the skin, which respond to sensations of warmth and touch, are stimulated by massage, warmth or water on the mother's whole body. These 'pleasant' sensations are transmitted to the dorsal column of the spine as well as the pain sensations, but the pleasant sensations can inhibit or reduce the transmission of some of the painful impulses.

In even simpler terms the pleasant sensations reach the brain faster and help to reduce awareness of the painful ones. As an added bonus, touch from massage and warm water immersion stimulates the hair follicles on the periphery on the skin, assisting in the production of pleasant sensations, partially or completely 'gating out' painful sensations.

The diagram below shows how a contraction can be perceived to be less intense than it actually is, because of the Gate Theory:

- The brain is receiving pleasurable sensations through the use of massage, water or heat, which overlap the pain sensations of contractions.
- Painful sensations arising from the uterus and pelvis travel along pain-receptor nerves to the spinal cord and then to the brain.
- The dorsal horn of the spinal cord runs along the entire length.
- Touch and warmth sensations on the mother's skin from the water travel along specific receptor nerves to the brain (via the dorsal horn).

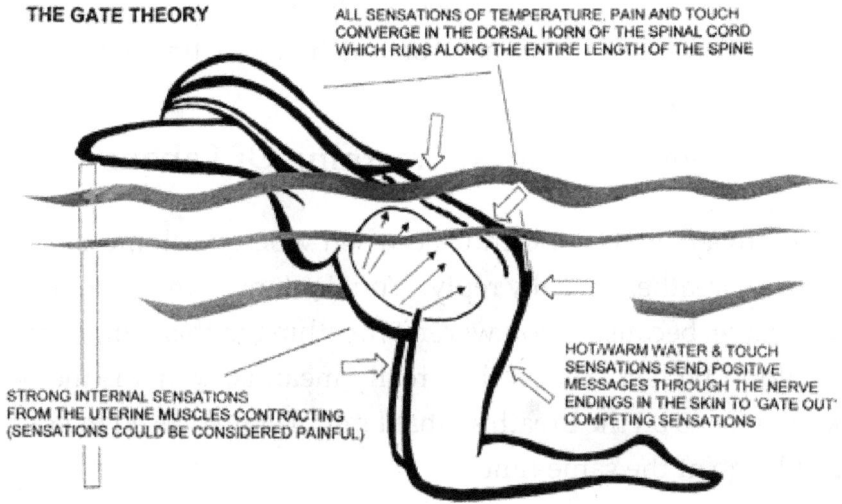

Other Internal And External Applications That Can Help During Labour

- Using Bach Flower Rescue Remedy or Australian Bush Flower Emergency Essence can help to keep the mind at ease and calm.

- Scented oils – buy a ready-made 'Labour Oil', or put a little lavender oil in cold-pressed apricot oil; the particular scents are intended to keep the body relaxed.

- Plain apricot oil for massage keeps the skin soft and lubricated, if being massaged for a long period of time. It can be applied to the perineum from time to time to assist with stretch and give of the skin when the baby comes through this tissue.

- Scented oils to burn in an electric burner (hospitals will not allow an open flame); having a pleasant smell in the room can make all the difference to how a person feels.

- Stereo for playing relaxing music. Music can assist greatly in creating the right mood for the occasion, although some people find any music too much of a distraction.

The Rhythmical Breathing Of Labour

It always makes me chuckle when women ask me to teach them to breathe. I usually reply, 'You don't need me to teach you to breathe, because if you weren't breathing at this moment you wouldn't be here.' What they really mean is, 'What is the best way to focus on the breath so that I might stay focused in labour and let go at the same time?'

The type of breathing that I recommend women and their partners use is one where a woman breathes in through her nose for the count of four, and out through her mouth for the count of six. If one contraction lasts approximately forty seconds, a woman can quite easily breathe in this rhythmical way four times during a contraction and the contraction would then be over. Because of this formula women tend to find the rhythm of their breath very quickly and discover that a contraction really lasts for such a short time; before they know it they are on their last cycle of 'in for four and out for six'. The time and contractions tend to pass very quickly this way.

Following is a diagram demonstrating the cycle of three breaths occurring while a contraction is taking place.

Natural Pain Relief From Water

From my own experience of three water births I can tell you I had a substantial reduction in labour pain upon being fully immersed in the water. This is the type of natural pain-relieving effect water can have. It is also the reason why women should be

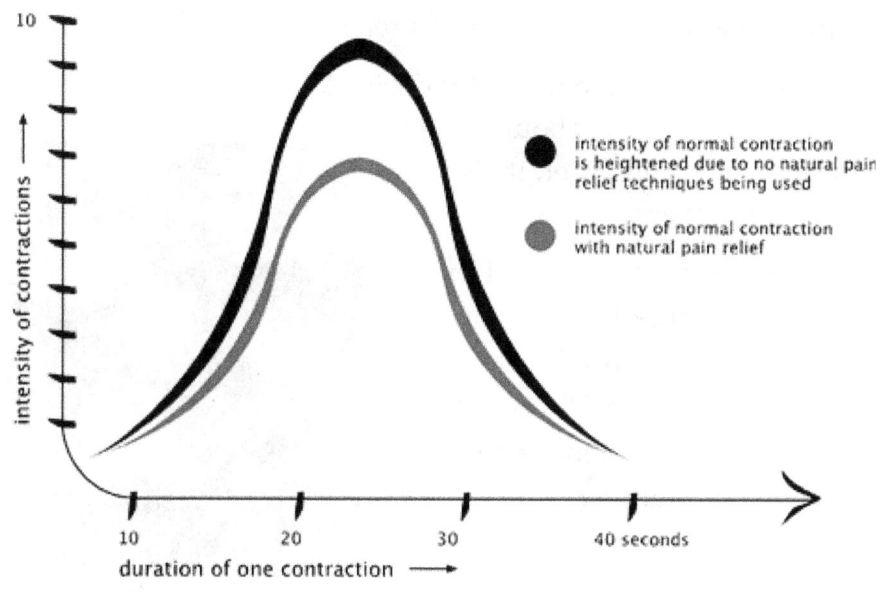
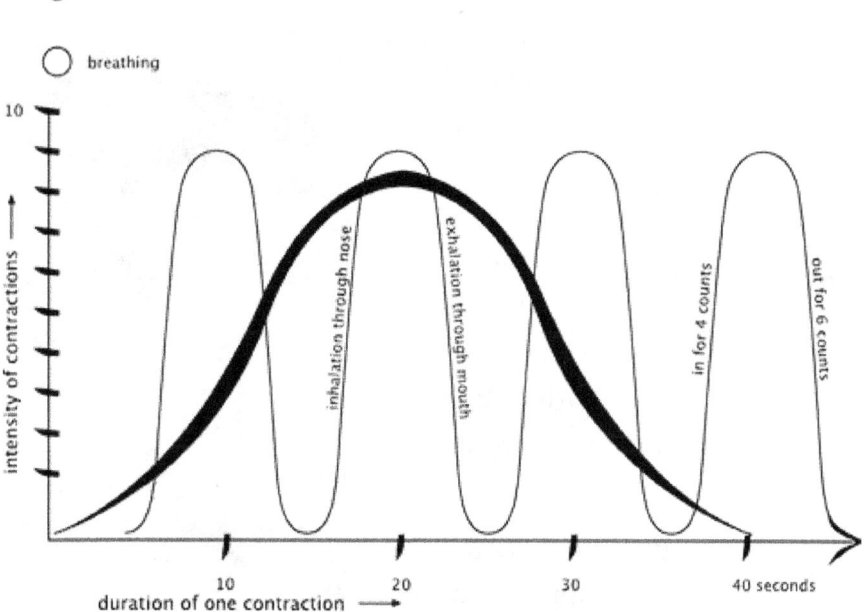

offered the use of a tub or shower, to assist them to cope with the contractions and remain calm and relaxed through-out labour.

Benefits of being in the water during labour. Being immersed in water during my labour not only assisted with pain relief, it also contributed in other ways:

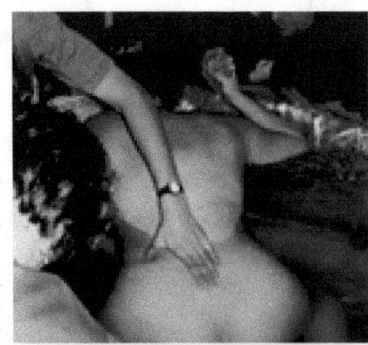

- The weightlessness I experienced due to being buoyant helped my tired, heavy body to be free and float and relax in between contractions, so I really could recover before the next contraction.

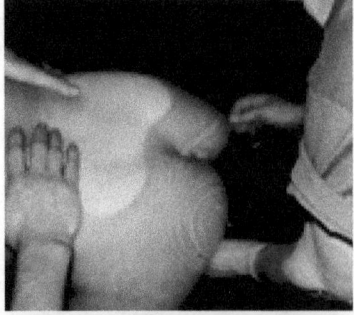

- The reduction in abdominal pressure due to lack of gravity (that is, the support of the water) helped my contractions to be really strong and efficient, which meant my uterine muscles worked effectively together. This resulted in more oxygenation to the uterine muscles, which assisted these muscles in opening the cervix in a shorter amount of time. Hence my labours were shorter.

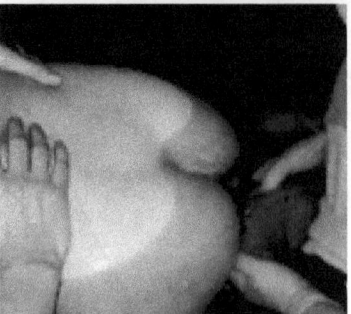

- The warm water helped me to feel really supported, comfortable and warm, which assisted me in labouring for

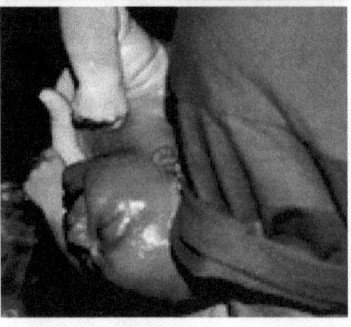

longer with no real reason to change positions due to discomfort.

- The sensation of the water helped my hormone/endorphin production to be stimulated and I went into the 'labour space' state, where I was calm and relaxed immediately upon immersion.
- Research indicates that you are also less likely to tear the perineum in a waterbirth.

If you plan on using a birthing pool it helps to do the following:

- Place a two-kilogram bag of fine cooking salt into your hot tub of water, which will stop you from becoming a prune! The salt will also help you to float and the perineum to stretch and give.
- To make your stay in the tub more comfortable, place a piece of soft foam (not rubber, it floats) on the bottom so your knees, feet and hands don't get sore and tired. This means you will be able to stay in the water for a longer period of time. Regularly filling up the tub with more hot water will help the tub to stay a really nice temperature and you won't get cold.
- It is a good idea to hire a birthing tub, rather than use a regular bath. You will have room to move in a birthing tub, whereas many people find a regular-sized bath far too uncomfortable during labour.
- Many people, especially those planning a homebirth, set up the tub some days in advance so that they can feel assured it is ready when they need it. However, if you decide to wait and set it up once labour has started, this would be a good job to delegate to a support person. Do make sure you have had a practice run at setting up a tub or pool that you have hired!

- An ideal depth of water is about seventy-five to ninety centimetres. However, I know one woman who jumped in the tub when it was only thirty centimeters deep and still being filled, finding it a perfect haven to let go and begin the work of strong labour.

- If you are lucky enough to have a home spa then you will have plenty of room to move in the water and the spa depth would be ideal. You may still need to place some foam at the bottom of the spa. Also, you should cover the filters of the spa so that no bloody mess (if there is any) gets sucked into the filter.

15

Hypnosis For Birth Preparation

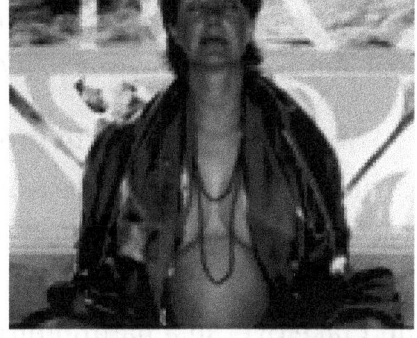

The Mongan Method

HypnoBirthing® is one of many programs available around the world. Created by Marie Mongan (from the United States), it is taught to pregnant women and their support people to prepare them for a relaxed, stress-free birthing experience. The philosophy teaches that when a woman is completely relaxed, well-informed and prepared both physically and mentally, she can experience a birth which is easier, more comfortable and potentially pain free.

I trained in Hypnobirthing® back in 2003 when it first came to Australia. The concept was simple offering self-guided relaxation with the premise that the more you practice and experience deep relaxation the easier it becomes. Hence, when a pregnant woman goes into labour she can easily go into a deep state of relaxation very quickly and hopefully stay in that place.

After using this method for a few years with my clients as a doula I realised my clients needed more so I went and trained as a certified advanced hypnosis practitioner. Hypnosis for Birth, my own program, enabled me to assist my clients to release fully prior to labour, any fear, stress or issues they had around their prior conditioning and beliefs about labour and giving birth. I could also assist my client to release birth trauma which is something that I foresaw was much needed for many of my clients and became an area of expertise and passion for me as the years went by. At this time I went into the record and recorded my hypnosis for birth scripts I put onto iTunes back in 2004 which to this day are still as relevant and powerful as the day I recorded them.

My Hypnosis for Birth program returns a woman to the art of birthing eliminating the fear of childbirth by teaching Grantly Dick-Read's theory of the fear–tension–pain cycle. It is also based on the belief that childbirth discomfort does not need to dominate and take over in a natural birthing situation. Hypnosis during birth utilises the fact that labouring women often want to just close their eyes and stay focused inwardly, internalising their feelings and emotions, in an altered state of consciousness. The labour/birthing hormones also assist with being able to allow the body/mind to let go and enter a deep hypnotic/meditative state with ease.

At one birth I attended (you can read the full birth story in the back of this book) I talked my friend down into a deep hypnotic relaxation by using keyword prompts and counting down. At this time she was in a hot tub, where she ended up spending a good four hours in the water labouring away. During that time she was in such a deep hypnosis induced state that she looked like she was asleep. She was in fact completely under hypnosis.

Between the contractions she would just sigh and breathe slowly in the most calm and relaxed way and during the contraction she would just breathe a little heavier. It really was the most amazing experience to watch. We (her partner and I) had the lights off and soft music playing in the background – it was truly beautiful. The most astounding thing about the use of deep hypnosis is the time warp that occurs. I remember my friend saying after the birth, 'I really wish I had more than half an hour in the tub as that was so relaxing!'

If you are interested in my own Hypnosis for Birth program, or any other programs that offer a similar approach, there are now practitioners around Australia and hundreds of practitioners in the United Kingdom and the United States. As a trained Hypno-Birthing® practitioner with an Advanced Certificate in hypnosis I offer many types of classes, workshops and private sessions around Australia (with amazing results being achieved – all via zoom). If you would like to explore this option further, go to my website, alabouroflove.com.au where you will find details of my hypnosis for birth program, including home study book.

Positive Birthing Affirmations

I have created the following affirmations based on my belief in the importance of pre-conditioning our brains to believe what we want them to believe. Our thoughts create our reality, so reciting these affirmations on a daily basis will make a big difference to the way you feel about yourself, your pregnant body and the birth ahead. I suggest you photocopy these pages and put them on the toilet wall, where you can read them daily. Say them out aloud too!

In preparation for labour, birth and parenting:

I totally trust that my body can do the job it is designed to do.

I put all fear aside as I prepare for the birth of my baby.

I am relaxed, focused and prepared for the birth of my baby. I am well-educated, strong and empowered for the birth ahead.

I am physically, mentally and spiritually ready for the birth of my baby.

I am ready for my new journey forward as a mother, provider and parent of this baby.

When I think about this birth, pleasant and exciting images come to mind and I feel blessed to be given this wonderful opportunity.

I am relaxed and happy that my baby is soon to be safe in my arms, physically present for me to smell, watch over and enjoy.

I am ready for a smooth and easy birth where I stay totally focused, surrendering to any sensations that come my way.

I feel confident, relaxed and ready for the birth ahead.

When I go into labour I will feel and experience each contraction as a single contraction only, just focusing upon that contraction in that moment. Nothing else matters.

In labour I will surrender and just let go.

I trust that the muscles of my body will work in complete harmony, to make my labour shorter.

On each and every contraction I will work on breathing in for the count of four through my nose, and out through my mouth for the count of six.

When I go into labour I will close my eyes and focus within, as this will help me to stay strong and focused and believing in my body's ability.

When I go into established labour, I will welcome each and every contraction as if it is a friend.

I will consciously release any tension I feel and let the natural instincts of my body take over.

During my labour I will trust and listen to my body, as it will guide me as to how I need to move and what I need to do.

I feel empowered enough to really state to the medical staff what it is I want and do not want during my labour.

16

What Women Need To Be Aware Of When Choosing To Use An Opiate Pain-Relief

I have included this subject matter as I feel it is important to provide accurate information about pain relief during labour, to allow women to make informed choices. I have been with women during labour when, after twenty-five to thirty hours of hard, established labour they have 'hit the wall' and opted for pain relief, understandably so. They then need to make an informed choice about their options. It is for this reason and this reason alone that I am including this information on drugs in a book where the focus is primarily about natural birth.

I would like to start by quoting from Dr Sarah Buckley's paper, 'Ecstatic Birth: Nature's Hormonal Blueprint for Labour'. Dr Buckley describes how using opiates during labour can result in missing out on some vital hormones – hormones responsible for how women respond and care for their baby after birth. She also describes how babies exposed to opiates in utero may later on look for the missing ecstasy they should have experienced during their birth.

In Dr Buckley's own words:

... as with oxytocin, use of opiate drugs will reduce a woman's own hormone production, which may be helpful if levels are excessive and inhibiting labour. The use of pethidine, however, has been shown to slow labour, more so with higher doses. Again we must ask: What are the psychological effects for mother and baby of labouring and birthing without peak levels of these hormones of pleasure and co-dependency? Some researchers believe that endorphins are the reward we get for performing reproductive functions such as mating and birthing; that is, the endorphin fix keeps us having sex and having babies. It is interesting to note that most countries that have adopted Western obstetrics, which prizes drugs and interventions in birth above pleasure and empowerment, have experienced steeply declining birth rates in recent years.

Dr Buckley goes on to say:

Of greater concern is a study that looked at the birth records of 200 opiate addicts born in Stockholm from 1945 to 1966 and compared them with the birth records of their non-addicted siblings. When the mothers had received opiates, barbiturates, and/or nitrous oxide gas during labour, especially in multiple doses, the offspring were more likely to become drug addicted. For example, when a mother received three doses of opiates, her child was 4.7 times more likely to become addicted to opiate drugs in adulthood. This study was recently repli-cated with a U.S. population, with very similar results. The authors of the first study suggest an imprinting mechanism, but I wonder whether it may be a matter of ecstasy – if we don't get it at birth, as we expect, we look for it later in life through drugs. Perhaps this also explains the popularity (and the name) of the drug Ecstasy.

What really amazes me is the fact that women will go through their entire pregnancy watching every bit of food and liquid substance that enters their body so that it does not harm their baby in any way, shape or form. Yet, when it comes to the labour and birth they do not hesitate to fill their body up with a concoction of opiates that affect not only the baby but also themselves. Why do women do this with so little thought and consideration of themselves or their baby?

Perhaps the answer to this question is that women in our culture fear birth so greatly that they will do anything to avoid having to go through labour and face the discomfort and pain associated with contractions. There is also the totally irrelevant argument that 'If you need a tooth extracted you would use pain relief so you don't have to feel it! Why wouldn't women do the same for childbirth?' My answer is that, unlike a tooth extraction, birth is a *totally normal process,* with natural hormones provided to help women cope and stay calm and focused amid pain that has a purpose.

Drug options for pain relief

In no particular order of preference I present the pros and cons of the various drugs available for pain relief during labour.

1. **Nitrous oxide – gas administered via a mask or mouthpiece**

Advantages:
- It is self-regulated, i.e. you decide on how much you have.

- It is self-administered: you decide when you want it.
- It has minimal effect on the baby.
- If you dislike it you can discontinue immediately.
- If you discontinue the effects wear off within a few minutes.
- A woman may feel as though she is very light and floating above the pain.
- A women can have it in the shower, the tub or walking around.
- It can be used during any stage of labour.
- It works within fifteen seconds of inhalation.

Disadvantages:

- It is only used when contractions are occurring.
- Some women dislike the feeling of being 'out of it'.
- It can cause women to vomit or feel nauseous.
- It is not perceived to be effective pain relief when used over a long period of time.
- It can cause difficulty with concentration.
- Women clench their teeth onto the mouthpiece and forget to breathe air or take it out in between contractions.

2. Pethidine – a narcotic drug

Pethidine is administered into the thigh or buttock via a needle.

Advantages:

- Stronger than nitrous oxide.
- Can help women sleep between contractions.
- Allows very tense women to relax.

- Effects can last up to two hours.
- Women may feel very warm and fuzzy, as if floating off in the far distance.

Disadvantages:

- It can cause a woman's breathing to slow down, and also her labour to slow.
- It crosses over the placenta and may depress the baby's respiration at birth.
- Baby may need oxygen at birth as it may be blue and oxygen-deprived.
- Narcan may need to be administered (via injection) to the baby to reverse the effects of the pethidine narcotic.
- Baby may be too sleepy to breastfeed for a considerable amount of time after birth.
- Some women completely 'freak out' on each and every contraction due to feeling really out of control.
- Some women still experience labour intensity, which can be exacerbated by pethidine.
- Some women vomit and feel very nauseated.
- Some women feel unable to communicate clearly, due to feeling so drowsy.
- It is not usually given during second stage, due to its effect on the concentration of the mother and it crossing the placenta to the baby.
- A vaginal exam (VE) is needed before it is administered (to determine 'how close' to birthing – but as discussed in Chapter 20, dilation does not necessarily follow a timeline and a vaginal examination could be perceived as unnecessary intervention).

- If a woman does not like the effect of the drug it can take up to two hours before it wears off.

3. Epidural

This is a local anaesthetic including cocaine derivatives, e.g. bupivacaine/Marcaine and, most recently, low-dose opiates. An epidural requires a thin tube to be inserted into the spinal cord between vertebra – it goes into the epidural space. The plastic tube is then connected to a pump so that a woman may keep topping herself up with the anaesthetic, so she no longer feels any sensations from the waist down, thereby anaesthetising the uterus, cervix and vagina.

Advantages:

- Does not make a woman drowsy.
- Allows a woman to sleep and rest if labour has been long. Usually gives total pain relief.
- Lowers blood pressure – useful if a woman has hypertension.

Disadvantages:

- Loss of bladder sensations so a woman has to have a catheter.
- If given too early in labour it can affect the baby's positioning, the rate of descent, the pressure on the cervix and dilation, which can stop altogether – resulting in a C-section.
- An intravenous drip is needed as blood pressure can suddenly drop – the extra fluid helps to maintain internal pressure.
- A woman is confined to bed – numb from the waist down.

- Baby will need constant monitoring with a CTG machine, which is strapped to a woman's body.
- Doesn't always work; this affects twelve per cent of women.
- It may partially numb the lower body – that is, one side of the body still feels every contraction, while the other half is blocked out. This affects three per cent of women.
- There is a chance of severe headache, lasting days or even weeks, if dura (spinal membrane) is punctured. This affects two per cent of women.
- Some women itch all over after having an epidural.
- Women lose the urge to push during second stage, hence the baby has to be assisted out (e.g. forceps or vacuum extraction, i.e. cascade of interventions).
- Some women will have extended numbing of the lower extremities that can last days, even weeks after the birth of their baby.
- Baby may need oxygen when born and may be slow to breastfeed or find it difficult to establish breastfeeding.

A note on 'walkabout' epidurals: Many people think these are a perfect solution, as you can theoretically be upright and mobile while also experiencing pain relief. However, they are forgetting that the opiate is still in their system and results in diminished feeling below the waist, often making it difficult to move effectively. Also, you can't go very far as you are often attached to a foetal monitoring machine. Some hospitals don't enable women to get off the bed at all when an epidural is in, because of litigation issues, such as falling over and injuring yourself.

17

Choosing And Educating Your Birth Support People

Being a support person for a woman in labour is the most rewarding, adrenalin-rushing, stimulating experience a person can go through. It can also be the most exhausting experience, both physically and mentally; it can take days to recover.

From my experience of attending many births, all totally unique and wonderfully individual, I realise there are some basic and fun- damental skills that birth support people need. It is not simply a case of turning up for a birth, saying a few soothing, encouraging words and a few hours later the labouring woman is ready to push and out flies the baby! I have listed the skills I feel are necessary to be a successful support person. This information is based on my experience and observations of what works and does not work.

Firstly, as a woman about to give birth, it is of the utmost importance that you ask yourself for what reason(s) you would like a particular person present at the birth of your baby. Secondly, make sure your support person/people are clear on what it is you are expecting from them. Drawing up a list of things you would like them to do is really important so that everyone is clear.

If you intend to have your partner with you, be really clear on what role you want them to play and exactly what you do and do not want them to do. This will prevent any unnecessary conflict when you are in labour – which can and does occur from time to time! If a woman thinks her partner is going to be an emotional mess and not cope at all, or if a partner does not want to be at the birth, consider other support options. Some people choose their mother or sister, whereas some couldn't imagine choosing family. Others choose women friends that they know will be positive and supportive of a good birth experience. Employing a doula – a professional birth support person – may be a good option. (The next chapter describes a birth doula in more detail.)

Your support person/people should read and think about the following points. It is also a good idea to discuss these points (and your birthing goals) with your support team.

- Intuition – as a support person, listen to your gut instinct about what the woman in labour is experiencing; only suggest things that are realistic to the moment, such as a change in position, place or environment, a shower, a back rub. Nine times out of ten it will be the right thing to suggest.

- Don't offer drugs because you think it looks like they are dying from the pain! Remember, you don't have the privilege of having all of the wonderful hormones on board, so sit back, and relax and support this woman in the best way you can.

- Expect the unexpected! Sometimes you will think it is all plain sailing when suddenly a woman gets blown off course. You may need to change course also. Or it may be over and done with very quickly, far faster than anyone imagined.

- You will need to give 110 per cent. A labouring woman demands your total mental, physical and emotional support, which can be stressful and exhausting, as well as rewarding!

- Be prepared to be awake all night and possibly still going through the next day. You may become a shift worker for a woman in labour. It is very hard to leave a woman in labour once you have been involved, because of the support you have given. Try to stay for the long haul if you have committed yourself.

- Ask yourself how you feel about giving massage, as it is quite possible that you will be doing it for hours on end. Most women in labour love massage, especially on the lower back. Note also that once massage has been initiated it is very hard for a woman to stop having massage, due to the Gate Theory of pain relief.

- Be assertive when necessary. Protect the woman from family members or medical staff that do not honour her need for privacy, peace or quiet. For example, it is very hard for a woman to focus on her contractions if a midwife is chatting away to someone – you may need to suggest that they be quiet.

- Talk the lingo. It really helps to have an understanding of the terminology that the hospital staff use. If you don't understand then ask staff to explain what they mean to you so you can relay back to the labouring woman what is going on. This allows her to keep focused on her labour state rather than having to engage in too much discussion with staff.

- Learn what to say when, and how to say it in a supportive way. Don't ask lots of questions or talk about rubbish as this can snap a woman out of labour. Know when you need to be a silent strength in the room, keeping the peace and quiet!

- Know how to find a soft, gentle tone in your voice to co-verbalise with the woman you are supporting. Help them to find their own individual sound. Really encourage deep, low sounds as these help women to push down vaginally and go to that primal space where they can open up and give birth.

- Understand the power of slow, controlled breath and the use of visualisations, deep meditation and relaxation to help a woman to open up and connect with her body.

- Help a woman to find the rhythm of breathing in for a count of four through the nose, then out for a count of six through the mouth.

Some Other Factors To Be Aware of As A Birth Support Person

- Serendipity. During the first part of labour a woman may be very chatty and excited about the whole idea of being in labour and having a baby. With this comes the opportunity to have a really good laugh and joke about all types of things. This can help a woman surrender early and go into labour more quickly, as she is relaxed and happy. Laughter also lowers the blood pressure, which can help tremendously.

- Offer one choice of drink, birth position, or type of food to eat – don't give her lots of choices or ask that she make decisions. Try not to ask lots of questions of a woman in labour as this forces her to come out of the labour space and therefore out of the primal part of her brain. For example, if you feel a drink is what is needed, just hold it up to her and she will either take it or shake her head to say 'No'.

- Beware of telling a labouring woman to relax! Some women in labour can relax in between their contractions while others feel the intensity of a contraction and the movement/pressure through the pelvis and lower back even when not contracting usually during OP (occipital posterior) presentation, baby's spine to mother's spine presentation. Nothing can be worse than being told to relax when you can't!

- Performance anxiety. When a woman is conscious of being watched or is asked repeatedly about contractions while in labour she can become self-conscious and start to feel very uncomfortable about the whole situation. This may occur if family members turn up unannounced and think birth is for general exhibition, or if a midwife or obstetrician stays in the room watching for progress. As a support person you can monitor the people in the room.

- Avoid clock-watching. Time has no relevance in labour. The reason the partners are asked to time the contractions is to give them something to do! After a while this can be stopped and a more productive and hands-on approach can be used. If you find yourself in a hospital room with a clock on the wall, take it off the wall and hide it where it can't be seen or cover it over with a cloth. Have all support people take off their watches as this stops any attempt to tune into what the time is. Clock-watching or continuously looking at your watch can be very distracting to a woman in labour. Remember that time has no relevance in labour, especially to a labouring woman. The only time that is important (at least in our culture) is when the baby is actually born.

- Dilation time has no rules. This is critical to remember. Many people believe that because it took two hours to reach one centimetre of dilation it is going to take another eighteen hours to get to ten centimetres. This is just NOT TRUE. Dilation does not obey mathematical rules! This is so important. Some women actually dilate and open within one hour. For most women, first time around the body can take a little longer to open because it has never done this job before. However, having said this, sometimes dilation is faster and sometimes slower, there really are no rules! So do not predict the length of labour based on the amount of dilation.

- Keep voices down. This will help a woman to feel at peace and relaxed with her surroundings, keeping her in the labour space.

- Out of pure love, often pain relief will be offered or suggested by the support person. It is not uncommon for a labouring woman's inexperienced support person/s or partner to suggest pain relief, because sometimes it is incredibly hard to see the person they love in so much pain and they want to turn it off and stop it. It is very important that this is discussed completely by all parties before the birth-day. I suggest that you make it quite clear on your birth plan and let your care provider know that if you want pain relief you will ask for it! And state, 'No matter what I say or do, do not ask me if I want it, I will ask you.'

- Work together as a team! If there is more than one support person then it is vital that you work together as a team.

Interacting With Medical Staff

Educate and empower yourself, your partner and your support people to ask questions if intervention is raised as a possibility by the medically trained staff. Every woman/couple has the right to make an informed decision on any procedure, and the facts must be presented so that they can understand the whole picture.

A woman and her partner need to ask questions of their medical care provider as soon as an intervention is suggested. I believe this is important, because if you don't question what is being suggested as soon as possible, circumstances may change, making it too late to clarify or discuss medical options. Women/couples may regret making an ill-informed choice when pressured and put on the spot by medical staff.

The Five-Minute Time-Out Rule

I suggest to women that every time an intervention is offered or recommended they request five minutes in private. Then the labouring woman and her support people/person (no medical staff present) can examine the options and discuss a possible change in plan. This ensures that an informed decision is made without the pressure of staff watching and listening. It is totally within your right to do this.

Questions a birthing partner, support person and labouring woman should ask

Below are some statements and questions you may need to use if medical staff want you to make a decision about something, or you do not agree with what is being suggested:

- Remember, you agreed we would not induce or rush this birth unless there was something wrong. Is something wrong?
- I ask that you honour our birth and be patient with what is occurring and not try to rush this labour, as I trust this labour is unfolding as it should.
- What is the medical indication here?
- I would really like a second opinion on this please.
- What harm is likely if we wait an hour or so?
- We'd like some time to think about it so we/I am not feeling pressured into making any rash decisions.
- Whoa, what's happening here?
- Is my wife in danger? If not we would like to stay with our birth preferences for longer and see how things progress.
- Is this baby in danger? If not then we would like to stay with our birth preferences for longer and see how things progress.
- What other options are there that we could consider?
- How would what you're suggesting affect my wife's labour?
- What effect could this have on the baby?
- Why do you feel this is necessary at this point?

- What indications do you see that tell you we should do this?
- My partner and I would really appreciate five minutes alone to discuss all of our options so that we can make an informed decision, without pressure from you.

18

Doula Support

In previous chapters I have briefly covered the benefits of having a midwife as your main care provider and also the reasons for which an obstetrician may be considered of value to your birth experience. In addition to having a midwife or an obstetrician you might also like to consider having a doula. In this chapter I would like to explain the role of a doula and describe the advantages women/couples gain through employing a doula. However, I must clarify before you read on that a doula is purely a birth support person and is not medically qualified. A doula is an additional person to your main health care provider.

What Is A Birth 'Doula'?

A doula is a birth assistant who provides continuous emotional support before, during and after the birth. They are not medically trained and are present during labour and birth to support the birthing woman. A doula can assist with massage, encourage a woman during labour and empower her through positive communication (verbal and non-verbal). A doula draws on her experience, knowledge and intuition about labour and birth.

Documented research is available which explains how the presence of a doula can shorten labour by two hours on average. This is just one positive aspect of having a doula. Other positive aspects found in a study of two thousand women are:

- Fifty per cent reduction in Caesarean rate. This is based on an assumption that 1000 women would need a C-section.
- Sixty per cent reduction in epidural request. This is due to the natural pain-relief methods being offered first and foremost, rather than a request for an epidural being made as the first response to pain.
- Forty per cent reduction of induction by oxytocin. Women who choose to have a doula often seek out natural methods to induce labour; hence there is less need for synthetic induction with a drip.
- Thirty per cent reduction in analgesia use (pethidine hydrochloride). The natural relaxation that women experience from massage, touch and positive verbal feedback allows a woman to stay very relaxed and calm, hence they experience less need for analgesic pain relief.
- Forty per cent reduction in forceps delivery. Women who have a doula are encouraged to stay calm and relaxed, upright, and off the bed, hence using gravity to assist the baby to move down through the birth canal.

The term 'doula' is Greek for a woman's slave or servant. During a birth a doula provides constant support and gives 100 per cent attention to a labouring woman and her partner. In a hospital setting medical staff might come and go, but a doula stays and only leaves a labouring woman if asked to leave by the woman she is supporting, or to have something to eat or go to the toilet.

A doula is often referred to as the 'missing link' in maternity care, because the medical care providers often don't have the time to offer the sort of care and comfort that a doula can, as they may be looking after other women at the same time. As well as this, medical staff often can't provide massage for the labouring woman for hours on end, or simply be in the birthing room as emotional support.

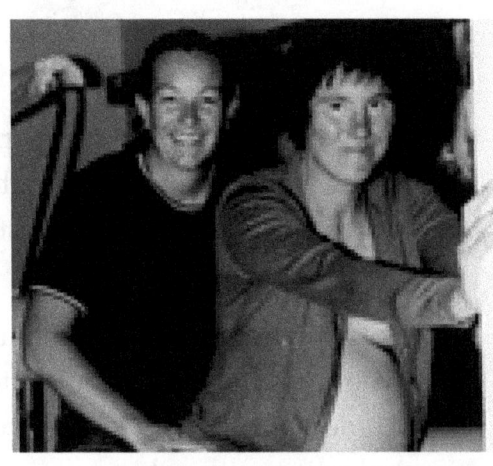

A concern that fathers often have when a doula has been asked to attend a birth is, 'What is the doula's role and where do I fit in?' In no way does a doula replace the partner – if anything a doula is present to reassure the partner that the birth is going how it should be and to keep the partner informed and educated about what is going on. This ultimately helps fathers to feel more relaxed and calm about seeing their partner in labour. I have attended many births as a doula where it was a team effort. The father rubbed the arms and shoulders while I massaged the back and the hospital midwife came and went, doing any medi- cal procedures.

One father described my presence during the birth like this:

Initially I was reluctant to have an 'outsider' at our birth. In hindsight, however, I am incredibly grateful to have had Gaby's intuition, skill, sensitivity and support, which she brought to every aspect of the birth. It took an enormous amount of pressure off me and allowed me to enjoy the whole experience in a way I don't think would be possible had we not had a doula.

Other feedback I have received from couples describes how they loved having someone else in the birthing room, someone they could trust and who was able to provide support and information about birthing. Partners often expressed sheer relief that I was there as an experienced birth support person, as they felt it took the pressure off them – they could relax more during the labour and the birth. Partners also felt they could handle seeing their partner in labour and were empowered to help them as best they could, following my lead in remaining very calm and positive at all times. This assisted the partner to appreciate what natural birth really looks like and to remain patient about the imminent birth.

The main doula benefits I see are:

- 'Continuity of care', which can start as early as four months into the pregnancy.
- Personal, specific and ongoing preparation leading up to the birth.
- Preparation of a birth plan.
- One hundred per cent personalised attention and commitment from a woman supporting you during your labour/birth.
- Assistance with personal issues at any time both before and after the birth.
- Access to information and classes available within the community relating to pregnancy, labour, birth and parenting.
- Information and help in making choices that directly relate to the labour, birth and post-birth period.

Choosing A Doula

When choosing a birth doula the most important thing is that both you and your partner feel comfortable with this person. Secondly, I suggest that you ask a doula to tell you about her beliefs and philosophy regarding birth. For example, below is what I believe as a doula, and I often give this out in a written form, as well as talking about it with women and their partners.

I believe that a woman is incredibly strong and powerful during childbirth, if she is given the right space, freedom and support from those around her at that time. This empowerment, belief and trust in her body comes from being educated about her choices and understanding totally what she wants when birthing her baby. It is the mother's and baby's right of passage to be brought into the world in the best possible way, and fear should play no part in that process. It is for this reason and this reason alone that I choose to support women and their partners during the lead-up to the birth and during the birth process on the birthday.

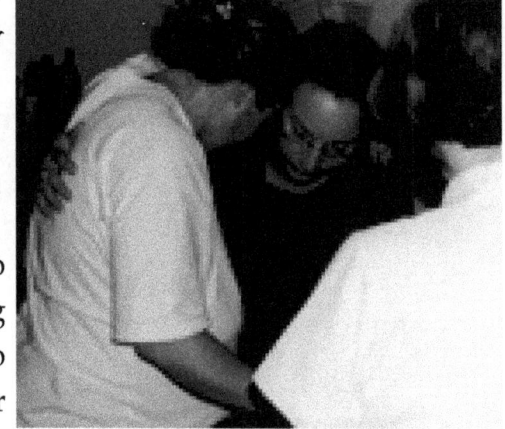

My aim as a doula is to support both the labouring woman and her partner so they may remember their baby's birth as a positive experience. Birth, after all, is a journey into Motherhood and Fatherhood, which can push both of you, physically, emotionally, mentally and spiritually, in every conceivable way possible. It is my job to guide you and support you into your new role as Mother and Father and to help you along on your journey.

I always provide all women and couples with the following information so everyone is completely clear about my role and the service that I provide, and so that there is no reason for anyone to be confused.

Please note that I am not a medically trained midwife, nor do I have the expertise to deliver a baby. But I will be at your birth to guide you through your journey. Should any decisions need to be made with regard to you, the birth, or about the baby, it will be your choice and final decision. I can help present all the necessary information with an unbiased opinion so that you can make up your mind given all the relevant information. I take no responsibility for the birth outcome, as I am there to massage you, quietly talk to you and help your partner, with the goal of helping you stay empowered and as focused as possible throughout the birth.

Other information that you may want to consider before deciding on the right doula for you:

- How many births have they been to previously?
- Is there a reference or contact phone number of a previous couple who you can talk to about their birth experience with this doula?
- How much does the doula charge?
- What does the fee include, for example: four visits leading up to the birth, attendance at the birth, etc.
- What you can expect during these visits?
- What form of training has she had?
- Has she ever worked at your place of birth?
- What is her role after the birth?
- What was your first impression?

Sometimes I really find it hard to describe exactly what I do at a birth and how one can put a monetary value on the work that a doula does. It is not easy to define, as it is so diverse: birth journeys are all so unique. I do know that when a woman pushes out her baby with a look of pure elation, ecstasy and relief and looks me in the eye and thanks me for assisting her, that this is what the work of a doula is about. Giving 110 per cent for hours on end to help a woman to have the birth she desires is why a doula provides the service she does.

Some of the birth stories at the end of this book are written by people for whom I have been a doula. Their stories help describe the role I have played in supporting their births.

19

EDD – Estimated Due Date, Give Or Take Two Weeks

I cannot emphasise enough that EDD stands for an ESTIMATED due date. Although women are obviously told that their EDD stands for an Expecting Due Date, there is sometimes an implication that they should be birthing on this day or before. Certainly, many obstetricians have policies that do not 'allow' women to go more than ten days 'overdue', counting from the EDD, which is only an estimate in the first place!

I hate this phrase EDD. It is often the first step in creating a performance anxiety as it can put into a woman's mind the idea that she has to go into labour sometime close to this date, and if she doesn't something is wrong with her body.

The problem lies not in the fact that the birth will obviously occur at some stage, but in how much pressure she is put under to have her baby within 'cooeee' of that estimate. What I have found during my research is that a great deal of pressure is placed on a woman who is over her EDD date, especially as she is then often referred to as 'overdue', when in fact her personal body/baby clock may not be ready for the birth. Women should probably only be described as 'overdue' when they are at forty-two weeks or more, as some babies need the whole forty-two weeks for gestation.

It is so important to remember that it is 'only an estimate' and it is very much a case of give or take two weeks. I know that every day over the estimated due date can feel like an eternity. However, as long as a baby is happy inside and all is fine, why rush this natural process – the baby has a hormone trigger that it releases when it is ready to be born. I know from experience how heavy a woman can feel, how swollen her feet can get and how huge and tired she can become as she gets close to birthing. It is hard not to opt for some assistance in getting things going, or give in to obstetric pressure to have an induction.

However, there are many reasons not to be induced, which I have addressed below. I do realise that sometimes it is necessary to be induced due to the baby being distressed or the placenta breaking down, and in these types of situations it is essential that a woman be totally open to what is being suggested by medical practitioners. (I want to make it clear that in my comments about avoiding an induction I am referring to women that basically opt to be induced because they are fed up and have had enough. I am also referring to the pressure that doctors can put on a woman who may be unaware that she has the choice to decline an induction if medical tests show her baby and placenta are doing fine.)

Women can experience an overwhelming amount of pressure from all types of people and sources, from the family doctor through to the stranger on the street, which can be very unsettling. Women often tell me that their friends are constantly phoning them to see if they have had the baby. Not to mention immediate family, as well as the in-laws (referred to as outlaws in some families!).

A simple solution to that problem is to take the phone off the hook and turn the mobile phone off. Another idea is to record a message on the answering machine, something like, 'Sorry we can't come to the phone right now, because we are resting and conserving our energy for the birth, which has not occurred yet, so leave your message and number so we can phone you when we have experienced the birth-day. Thanks for phoning.'

If your friends and family keep coming to the door, put a note on the door that states: 'Mother-to-be sleeping, under no circumstances are you to knock unless it is a real emergency. Thank you for your understanding and patience.'

Another area of stress and pressure could actually come from a woman's chosen obstetrician. It is unfortunate but true that they may make the decision for the woman that the baby needs to come out, without any real medical indications. I have heard stories over the years about the real reasons behind women being persuaded and coerced into being induced (for example, on the day of a general checkup appointment which fell on the EDD or after the EDD by a few days).

Reasons for inductions given to some women by medical care providers (some of which may be relevant in some situations) sound something like this:

- *'Your baby is too big to it through your pelvis.'* The doctor is suggesting that inducing early will mean a slightly smaller baby but a good midwife will show you positions that can really open up your pelvis – not to mention the effect of relaxin, which is designed to make your pelvis flexible.

- *'Your amniotic fluid is getting really low.'* I have been led to believe that amniotic fluid replenishes itself every day, hence it is unlikely to be too low for it is always reproducing!

- *'I think this placenta is starting to shut down.'* Ask the doctor, what was the medical test performed to indicate this? Some doctors instil fear that the placenta will degenerate after the EDD, without checking that particular woman's placenta. Many placentas function perfectly fine up to forty-two weeks.

- *'I think we need to get things moving along.'* If a woman has been labouring away for a few days but is still in 'Warm Up' mode with the odd strong contraction, she may be convinced to have an induction. A good alternative might be to get into the bath or shower, with dim lights, and try some hypnosis or do some visualisations of going into labour with strong, dynamic contractions.

- *'If you don't let me induce you, you are putting your baby at risk.'* The question to ask is HOW? What evidence suggests this? If you are not given a straight and honest answer use your own discretion as to which way to proceed.

- *'You may never go into labour at this rate.'* On what basis can a doctor make this negative assumption, one which again starts the performance anxiety loop? As far as I am aware, ALL women will spontaneously go into labour, unless they are carrying a baby with spina bifida or similar condition.

Not all of the above are genuine reasons for an induction, and indeed most are based in fear, rather than a sense of trusting the body. If a woman finds herself being pressured in this way it would be a good idea to seek a second opinion straight away. If her suspicions are right, the doctor's reasons for induction are perhaps just to get the birth out of the way, before the weekend or a planned holiday. (This is not just an urban myth!)

It is also easy to get a medical check on the baby and the placenta by arranging for a non-stress test. This is a non-invasive test where several of baby's measurements are recorded for half an hour, to clarify that the baby is still doing fine inside. This NST can be done daily, or every second day, past the EDD. Even if you are homebirthing, your GP or local maternity hospital can organise for you to have this test if you are concerned about your baby or your placenta's condition.

I suggest to women that they ask for more time, if that is what they feel is the right thing to do. Try to relax and give yourself permission to have the time you feel is necessary to further prepare for your labour and birth. Try not to be anxious or uptight or worried you have made the wrong decision. There may also be some small issues you still need to ponder and clarify in your own mind before your body feels free to go into labour.

Getting Labour Kick-Started
– Some Natural Stimulus Ideas

There are many natural stimuli that you can explore to assist you to go into labour. The following are a few that have been very successful for various women that I have met, and some are methods I have personally used.

- Having sex with male ejaculation (the sperm is a natural prostaglandin) helps to soften the cervix and prime the birth canal. A female orgasmic experience is equally as important as this gets the pelvic floor and surrounding muscles contracting and stimulated. The more orgasms and ejaculations experienced the better!

- Nipple stimulation can be very beneficial. It needs to be continuous and ongoing for five minutes at a time with a five-minute break, over one hour. Any form of sucking, pulling and stimulating through rubbing is required to simulate the release of oxytocin, which can cause the cervix to start softening and thinning out, effacing. This can be tedious and make your nipples/breasts sore if tender, so it is suggested that you use an oil or cream that is suitable to put on your nipples. Apricot oil or pawpaw cream would be ideal (or feed your toddler, if you are still breastfeeding another sibling).

- There are homeopathic remedies that can assist a woman to release any pent-up emotions or fears surrounding birth. A woman would need to see a homeopath for the right blend to work through any possible emotional blocks.

- Acupuncture can be very successful, however a woman should seek out a qualified acupuncturist with experience of inducing women into natural labour.

- There is nothing like a good spicy curry to get a woman going. It works on the premise that when the lining of the stomach wall is stimulated with hot, spicy food and the digestion process is intensified, the nerve endings around the uterus will follow its lead and start contracting.

- The same can be said for any spicy food or castor oil – they work by upsetting the stomach lining, which can trigger the uterus to start contracting. However, it is important to know the true effect of ingesting castor oil is that it works as a laxative and generally gives women a dose of the runs! But hey, that could be considered a small price to pay as often women do go into labour and spend a good part of labour on the loo anyway! Look on the bright side, you are less likely to do a poo during your labour if it is all emptied out first! (A small caution about overdoing castor oil is warranted here. Seek out a midwife to help you take the castor oil. Don't overdo it and once taken allow it time to work. More than two lots within four hours could be considered too much.) What to do: Take one tablespoon of castor oil, followed by an orange juice to stir things up. This process can be repeated up to three times over a day. It will usually only require one or two tablespoons and you're off and running, literally! If things have not started by then, maybe you are just not really ready, or you have a stomach lining made of steel!

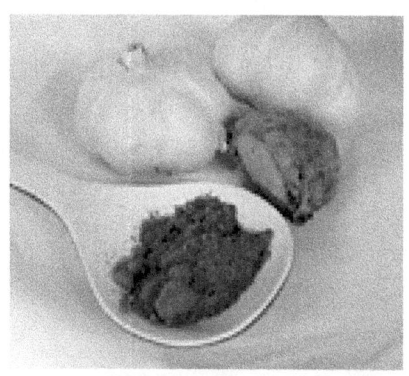
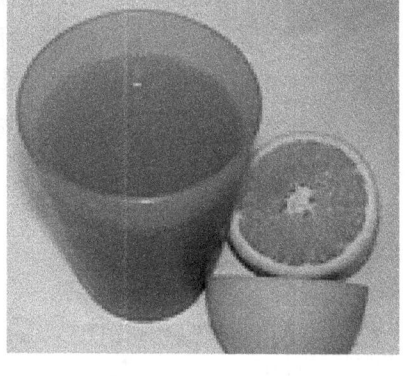

- For some women, exercise can provide the necessary overload on the body to get them in labour. Walking is ideal, as is getting into water. On a few occasions I have had women come to my aquatic exercise classes to get things moving along. Be active and move if that is what you feel is right for your body. If you are going to a public pool to attend an aquatic exercise class or swim laps make sure your waters have not broken,

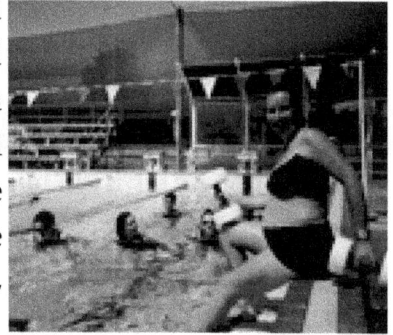

as this means you have lost your natural protection and plug that stops any unwanted bacteria and germs from the swimming pool getting up inside. Swimming in the ocean is fine.

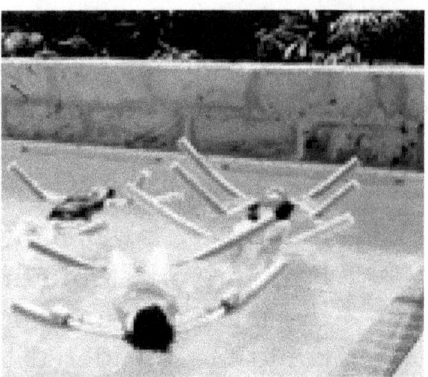

- The power of visualisation is one of the most amazing and powerful tools that everyone has access to. If a woman can just sit and let her body go into a deep relaxation or meditative state, in which she visualises her body opening up and her

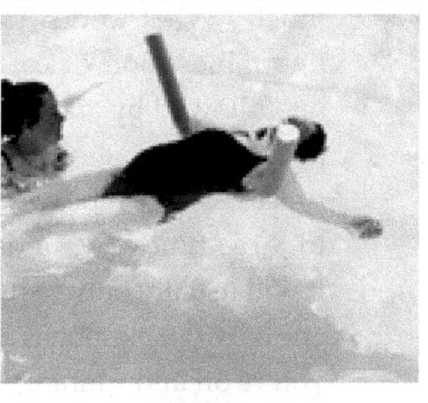

muscles contracting, the chances of going into labour spontaneously will be increased tenfold.

- There are many types of deep relaxing music available that can assist you to stay relaxed and positive, mindful that your imminent birth will occur when the time is right for you.

- Drinking raspberry-leaf tea can aid some women to go into labour, especially if their uterus is sensitive to contracting after a cup has been drunk. However, if a woman has been drinking two to three cups a day from week thirty-five, it is unlikely that she is going to go into spontaneous labour from drinking the tea. Women often drink raspberry leaf tea in late pregnancy as it helps the uterine muscles to tone up so they may work efficiently and effectively when in labour.

20
What Do You Do When Labour Starts?

A lot of women ask me the following questions, so I would like to respond to these questions in the hope that it will help women to gain a better understanding of the early stages of labour, particularly if you are pregnant for the first time.

What do I do when I go into labour?
How will I know that I am really in labour? How does labour actually start?
When do I need to ring the hospital? (If you are going.)
How long do I have after my waters break, before I go into the hospital?

Well, here goes. How most women go into labour is not a simple question to answer, as the thing to remember here is that everyone is different, so I am writing from my experience of what I have observed first hand. Every situation was unique and totally different from the previous birth I attended. There are always exceptions to each scenario, so I am providing the information below in general terms.

One thing that usually occurs even before the niggles start or the waters break is the presence in a woman's undies of the 'bloody show', which is the mucus plug that seals the cervix starting to come away. It basically means things are warming up and thinning out 'up there'. The mucus plug can actually start to come away as early as two weeks before a woman's estimated birth-day. However, when a woman is in labour it tends to be a very runny mucus that is often tinged with blood or a brown (old blood) show. There is not a lot of blood, it is more mucus than anything else. With the release of the plug the birth canal begins effacing (or thinning out) from a heavy, thick wall to a paper-thin wall. As a result of all this activity the cervix will also start to dilate. Some women may be as much as two centimetres dilated before they have even experienced a contraction.

Many women will go into natural labour with their membranes (water sac) breaking suddenly, or the membranes may not break till much later in the labour, or even not until the baby comes through the perineum during the final stage. Some women will start with a dull ache in their lower back that slowly begins to get a little stronger as the hours pass, while others will feel a period-type pain that starts as a niggle, then comes and goes in a rhythmic wave, strengthening as time goes by.

Birthing Contractions (The 'Real Thing') Or Braxton Hicks Contractions?

One of the main differences between 'birthing contractions' and 'Braxton Hicks contractions' is that a Braxton Hicks tends to be a sensation of all-over hardening of the abdominal area, like the baby is pushing its body outwards as hard as it can. I remember this sensation as being like someone turning my abdominal area into a basketball, as it felt so hard and round in a short space of time. Accompanying that sensation was often a discomfort right down in the lower abdominal area. Many women feel Braxton Hicks during their pregnancy, while others do not. This has absolutely no bearing on whether or not a woman's uterus will or will not contract properly when she goes into labour. It is true that a Braxton Hicks is like a warm-up contraction of the uterus, in which it hardens from about thirty seconds to about two minutes. Some women have them all the time but don't feel it when they do, often because they do not realise what they are, or they are not focusing in on the different changes and sensations of their body.

A birthing contraction, on the other hand, is more rhythmical and will generally start with a wave-like sensation which starts off mildly building in intensity till it peaks and then eases off. These contractions being initially further apart in distance and getting closer together as time goes by.

As I mentioned earlier, one of the main benefits of going into labour naturally is that women get to experience a 'warm up' in which they can prepare themselves for the imminent birth.

A contraction generally lasts for about forty seconds in duration. During this time a woman can breathe in and out slowly three times, taking approximately forty seconds, by which time the contraction will be over. I would like to mention here that nature has been incredibly kind to (most) women by giving them a wonderful break in between contractions. This allows for sleep (catnaps), deep relaxation, floating (if in water) or to have a drink or eat some food, or poop or pee if needed. A lot of the best labour work comes from utilising the time in between the contractions, so that when a contraction takes place a woman is mentally and physically prepared and ready to surrender to it.

To Break or Not To Break The Membranes, That Is The Question

So you have started labour and you have possibly moved into the hospital. Now a key question to ask is, 'Should the membranes be broken?' A woman's labour may start with or without the membranes breaking. I had the lucky experience of giving birth to two babies with my membranes intact, as they just did not break till my boys' heads emerged from my perineum. This does occur from time to time, as long as the birth attendants don't interfere with them and feel the need to break them.

Having the membranes broken artificially, 'just because they should be', or 'because it will speed things up', or 'for no real reason', is a woman's choice. I have heard of many stories where a routine vaginal examination was performed with a glove that had a little hook on the end of the fingers and the membranes were broken without the knowledge or consent of a woman!

My third birth with Jarrad was with my membranes intact, and it was only two hours of established labour. Having the membranes intact does not always mean you are going to labour for a long time! Neither does having your membranes broken assure you of a faster labour. Yet a common explanation as to why medical care providers want to break the membranes is to get things moving along and speed labour up. What's the hurry?

Women in labour need to take it upon themselves to decide if this is really necessary or not. Often the watery sac/membranes in front of the baby's head cushions it down into the perfect position on the cervix and after a period of time the membranes will naturally break. So this is a good reason not to interfere, perhaps also explaining why the membranes don't always break immediately when you go into labour.

However, having said all of that, if a woman does have the urge to push and her waters are bulging, she may feel them hanging down. At this stage it could be time to have them broken, as they have done their job and cushioned the baby's head down into the correct position on the cervix. Sometimes they don't break at this point because the membranes are so tough, like strong heavy-duty plastic/film. If they were left they would still eventually break at some point, probably as the head comes out, or maybe the membranes would be intact around the baby. (In times gone by this was considered to be very lucky!)

If your membranes do break and you are at home you can still stay at home and really give yourself a chance to go into labour in your own space, environment and time. The only difference is that you need to make a mental note at what time the membranes broke, so you can relay this information at a later time to the hospital staff. Some hospitals will have you on the 'stop watch' and give you between twenty-four to thirty-six hours, depending on the hospital, to go into established labour when the membranes have broken. This is one of the reasons couples are asked to head on into the hospital as soon as the membranes have broken, regardless of whether labour has started. The only problem with this is the anxiety and stress a woman can feel can be exacerbated, and she may feel an overwhelming pressure to start labour. If labour does not start the catecholamines may elevate, as does the performance anxiety, in which case a woman may never go into labour naturally.

Yes, it does feel like the pressure is on when this occurs. The reason the hospital staff want women to go into established labour within this time frame is to avoid the risk of infection. If a woman has not gone into labour before the twenty-four to thirty-six-hour mark, antibiotics may be given as a precautionary measure. Women in this situation need to watch out and not get caught up in anxious thinking or focusing on the possibility of getting an infection. This prospect alone can cause undue stress and impatience with one's body, which in some cases means a woman may never go into proper labour, due to a heightened sense of tension being present (refer to the effect of hormones such as adrenalin mentioned in earlier chapters as well as the fear–tension–pain theory).

Some hospitals have a policy that if your membranes have broken you are not allowed to enter into a hot tub, while other hospitals do not see this as an issue. Research does suggest that going into public swimming pools once the membranes have gone is not advisable, because there are so many foreign bacteria which could pose a problem. However, the small private bath at your home or at the birthing centre or hospital will only contain your bacteria, which you have released into the water, posing no real problem at all apart from a small risk of cross contamination.

How The Membranes Usually Depart The Body

When a woman's membranes do go they will often go as a huge gush, hitting the floor in a flood. A common urban myth is that if this occurs in a shopping centre you should be able to get your shopping for free. I think this is an excellent idea, but then again I am not a shop owner having to pay for the cost of a woman's grocery items. Another suggestion that I have heard is to 'accidentally on purpose' drop a drink container (or a jar of pickles!) on the floor so that it is not so obvious that the membranes are leaking down your legs … Membranes breaking while shopping has occurred on many occasions, much to the horror of some women who have just left the shopping trolley in the aisle and raced out, leaving a big wet patch followed by a trail of drips!

A less dramatic way for the membranes to depart is to trickle, and trickle they will, with every movement and contraction alike. I always recommend that a woman should go straight to her nappy collection, disposable or cloth, whichever takes her fancy, and tuck them into her undies. If a woman chooses just to stay with her maternity pads, she will find that she will have used her entire packets before she has given birth. Maternity pads are an expensive way to soak up your membranes – cloth nappies or disposables should definitely be considered. Besides, who is going to know or see you, except other women in the same position as you walking the streets or the corridors of the hospital in labour.

Reasons to stay at home to really allow your labour to get going

As a result of going into hospital too early, 'performance anxiety' can become an issue because a woman may feel extra conscious that she is being observed and watched by staff, as they establish some idea of what is happening. This can be detrimental to her progress at this time, as she may be very aware that she is not far enough along into any rhythmical warm-up or experiencing established labour type contractions. The amount of pressure felt from the care providers, family and sometimes the partner can often cause a huge amount of stress. As a result the catecholamines build up, and the body and the muscles of the uterus tense up. Hence, the body slows down or stops altogether.

It is extremely common for women to go to hospital in fairly early labour, thinking it is all happening, only to find their labour seems to stop and they are sent home again. For some women this can make them feel like naughty schoolgirls who haven't done their homework properly – for most women the implication is that their body isn't working properly. Again, performance anxiety can have a disastrous effect on the progress of a natural labour.

Induction at this point may sound like the best option, and it may appear an easy way out of this situation (by not needing to go home again, as the labour is 'augmented'). But staying at home, if at all possible, has a huge advantage for women in the early stages of labour, as they can relax and not be constantly reminded that the clock is ticking! They also have the freedom to move about the house, going wherever they feel like going or just resting, sleeping on their own bed or doing whatever they feel like. This kind of freedom and non-restrictive environment can be very beneficial, and in turn will assist a woman to remain relaxed and go into labour when the time is right for her, without pressure from others. By staying at home a woman can also feel extra safe in her familiar environment.

Some women will actually be in light warm-up labour for many hours (possibly days) before they start to feel the urge to put their head down, close their eyes and really focus inwardly, indicating more established labour. During the warm-up stage women are often very bubbly and talkative and happy to move about.

When a woman starts into established active labour she will generally want to work on contractions with her eyes closed, head buried in a pillow, or leaning against a wall in an upright position. Women generally know that they are in established labour as when a contraction comes on they will want to stop talking, focus inwardly, and move in some way perhaps sway their pelvis from side to side, while concentrating on breathing.

At this point it is a good time to consider where in the house a woman may want to go to get comfortable, so she can start assisting her body to stay relaxed and calm, and move into a more dynamic rhythm with her contractions.

At this early stage of labour a bath is usually not a good idea. When building up to established labour, women may find that being fully immersed in a tub of hot water is so relaxing that it actually slows labour down to next to nothing, which is not what a labouring woman wants to happen. The shower, on the other hand, can assist in making the shift from the warm-up stage of labour to the more focused established labour.

As my friend Liz explained to me: 'A warm shower on my back masked the incredible increase from early to established labour – I got out of the shower and realised "kapow"– it's really here now.'

One of the previously mentioned passive/active labour ideas might also be an option in the early part of established labour, such as sitting on the fitball rocking through the pelvis, or leaning over pillows on the bed with hot packs on the lower back and pubic area.

At some point, when labour has really started to progress, if she is planning to birth at hospital a woman may want her partner to phone the hospital to let them know that she has gone into labour. However, do be aware that when this call is made often the midwife on the other end of the phone wants to talk to the labouring woman, to see if she is really in labour. If you really are in labour the last thing you feel like doing is talking to someone on the phone and answering questions! I guess this could be a woman's simple gauge. If you can talk on the phone you are not far enough along into labour to head into the hospital. If you can't talk on the phone because you are working hard on the contractions as they come, you are ready to go into the hospital!

Be aware that talking on the phone to anyone is the surest way to snap any woman out of that lovely labour state. A support person or partner is quite capable of answering all the necessary questions that are asked and can explain the body language exhibited when a woman has a contraction.

Any good midwife will usually suggest that if there have not been any complications with a woman's pregnancy that she stay at home for as long as she can, and labour where she feels comfortable and relaxed in her own surroundings. This can and does help a woman to really let go and allow herself to get into established labour.

If a woman does venture into the hospital too soon and she is not really in established labour, the transition of leaving the lovely home setting and moving into a white-walled sterile environment might be the reason for a labour shutting down and grinding to a halt. Being aware of this phenomenon is a good reason to stay home a little longer.

Some women who go into hospital too early are asked to go home and come back when labour is established. If this happens to you, then do go home! The unlucky ones who are asked to stay in the hospital often complain, in hindsight, that they felt very tired due to all the medical checks throughout the night and day, general hospital hustle and bustle, hospital noise, not to mention the sound of babies crying through the night. So, when they finally went into labour they were exhausted, with little to no energy due to being so tired. This type of scenario is not at all conducive for a woman who would like to labour naturally and experience a natural birth.

In the hospital – the VE (vaginal examination) – is it really necessary?

When a woman does make the shift from home to the hospital she may find that labouring away for hours in a tiny room with shared shower/toilet facilities is not what she had in mind, and it may make her distracted and uneasy. These types of feelings should be avoided at all costs. Added to this could be a sense of not being able to go anywhere, and the realisation that sooner or later a vaginal examination – or internal, as they are often referred to – is going to take place. This is often mentioned upon arrival at the hospital just in case a woman has forgotten!

An internal examination is something that occurs upon arrival at just about all hospitals in Australia. There are, of course, exceptions to the rule. For example, when a woman labours very quickly and starts to push the baby's head through the birth canal unexpectedly, an internal is not recommended. Or if a woman states in no uncertain terms that she is not going to have one, she may be able to put off having any, providing there is nothing holding the baby back or the woman from pushing the baby down the birth canal.

The thought of walking into a hospital and having a total stranger do an internal is a little off-putting for a lot of women, to say the least. This is why it is a really good idea to go into hospital when you are really in established labour, so at this stage it may seem less of an ordeal to actually have a VE (if you still want to have one) and hopefully will not affect how dilated you are. This, of course, can depend on who does the VE, if it is done gently with respect and with what intention they do it.

Ina May Gaskin, writes:

I remember a birth that taught me that a rough and uncompassionate pelvic examination can reverse a mother's cervical dilation. I was attending the labour of a first-time mother, who developed a fever. It soon became evident that it was caused by a bladder infection. Although she had reached seven centimetres of dilation, she was not moving past that point. I decided that I should transport her to a hospital. When we arrived at a hospital in Nashville (with her dilation still at seven centimetres – I checked just before we got there), her care was assigned to an obstetrician who was rather sullen and unfriendly in his manner. With no pleasantries of permission, he examined her internally so roughly that she cried out in pain – a reaction she had not had during my previous examinations. He muttered that her cervix was only four centimetres dilated and left the room for a few minutes. While he was out, I confirmed that her cervix was four centimetres dilated with my own examination. I was sure it was his painful, rough examination that closed her cervix that much.

On two occasions within the hospital system I have supported women who have said in no uncertain terms 'No Way' to internal examinations, and have got away with labouring and birthing naturally and not having one single internal. So, you ask, 'Why is it necessary?' The midwives are instructed by the hospital to perform them on all labouring women upon being admitted to hospital, so they then have an idea of how dilated a woman is upon arrival. They then use this dilation estimate as a gauge that basically goes like this:

According to the textbooks, a woman is supposed to dilate at one centimetre per hour, and if you are not dilating to that plan, something is just not going right! My thoughts on this are that this so-called formula does not take into account each woman's unique and individual body.

Be aware! Dilation has no rules – it is just an estimation of what the body could be doing, which does not take into account that everyone is different! You do have a right to say 'No' to an internal if you do not want one. No one can make you have one if you really feel strongly about this.

Another point to note is that what often occurs after an internal is that a midwife will tell a woman she is only two centimetres dilated. Now, if a woman has been labouring for six hours, for example, and she hears this, she starts to do the labour math in her head, based on what the books say, and she then starts to feel emotionally beaten, not to mention mentally lost. Telling a woman she is not really progressing does nothing for her self-esteem, not to mention her belief in herself and her body, or to empower a woman to trust that all is OK. Performance anxiety again could very much come into play.

This false belief about dilation can be very disempowering for women and can totally shatter their ideas about birthing naturally in an instant. If a woman, on the other hand, is told after an internal: 'Well done, you are doing a wonderful job of opening up, your body is working beautifully' she may jump from four centimetres dilation to ten within the hour. A positive mental attitude can really be that inspiring, causing the physical body to respond accordingly. As simple as this seems, a positive comment suggested to a woman in labour can influence her greatly in the way she feels, giving her the strength to believe she is capable of continuing, in a trusting way, where she feels that every contraction has a purpose – that purpose being the opening up of her body, which inevitably is getting her one step closer to meeting her baby.

Our thoughts really do create our reality, so what is it that you are thinking and feeling? When we put a clear enough request forward a response will follow in kind, that's the way it works! Trust in this process as it really does work.

The point I am trying to make is that every woman has a choice as to whether they do or do not have an internal examination. If they decide they are going to, because they want to know how dilated they are, I suggest that a woman has a midwife tell her the number of centimetres she is between one and ten, with no other dialogue between the two people concerned. Use of the word 'only' in part of her dialogue can have such a great impact on a woman during labour. This way a labouring woman can interpret the information how she likes. It is like saying, 'Is the cup half full or half empty?' It is up to an individual to decide.

On a more positive note I feel the following story is really worth reading, as it again reinforces how important the connection is between our thoughts and our body, and how the two are interconnected. This story is from *Ina May's Guide to Childbirth*:

After a while I checked her internally to see how open her cervix was. She said, 'I just want to open up and let this baby out.' As she spoke these words, her cervix yawned open another two centimetres beneath my fingers. Now I was experiencing behaviour that I didn't normally see, since I had never heard a woman express the wish for her cervix to open while I had my fingers on it to confirm that it was happening. Pretty fancy I thought, to be able to tell your body exactly what you want to happen and have it comply.

21
Established Labour

Early established labour is the next stage of the labour journey. Labour can be compared to an endurance event, during which some women experience the feeling of 'hitting the wall' at some time. It is at this time that women really need their birth support person/people to help and assist in any way they can, to get a woman through this stage. The average length of a labour for a first baby is anywhere between twelve and twenty hours in duration. However, I was an exception to this rule, as were many other women who I have attended.

We realise that the first baby arrives rather more slowly than others, and also that it entails possibly more hard work in the second stage of labour; but there is no necessity for any more discomfort and certainly no reason to be afraid of the arrival of the eldest child than the birth of its brothers and sisters.
Grantly Dick-Read.

Being in established labour can be mentally and physically challenging for a woman, and if the labour has been going on for a long time she may be thinking that her body is not opening up very quickly, or, worse still, that nothing is happening at all.

Massage, Bach Flower drops under the tongue (Rescue Remedy) or Australian Bush Flower Emergency Essence) and giving lots of verbal reinforcement and positive verbal stimuli/suggestions are exactly what is needed. If a woman in labour is constantly being told she is doing a fantastic job, that her body is doing really well, her body is opening up beautifully, etc., a woman's body will respond accordingly, which could be paramount at this point during a labour. Do not underestimate our ability to physically create what we want through our thought processes.

During established labour a woman may feel like she needs to move about and change positions regularly to assist in getting the baby's head down. When I have sometimes thought to myself, 'I don't think this woman has any reserves of energy to move about', I have been totally wrong.

Our thoughts really do create our reality, so think positively and believe in you!

Women have the most amazing strength and ability with the production of adrenalin towards the transitional stage of labour, and can move and do what feels right for them without any hesitation. They will often pace and walk in between contractions just before feeling the urge to push. As if out of nowhere comes a rush of adrenalin to get a woman recharged, alert and ready to start pushing the baby's head down and through the cervix and into the birth canal. (This is a positive result from the adrenalin rush occurring at an appropriate time.)

Food And Drink In Labour

When the uterus is contracting with such a dynamic force, a huge amount of blood is shunted to the working muscles time and time again, contraction after contraction. The uterine muscles of the body are like any other working muscle in that they need a constant supply of fuel to keep consistently contracting over a period of time. Hence, small snacks are ideal, and I emphasise small snacks, as these will ultimately keep the muscles working with full intensity and ability. If you try to have a large meal or sandwich you may find that it comes back up, or it will sit in the stomach for ages, as digestion of food during labour is not the body's priority. Labour is a much more important function at this time.

A woman should be given the opportunity to snack on small amounts of complex carbohydrate-rich foods, such as bananas, dry biscuits, multigrain bread and plain rice, all of which are perfect for a slow release of energy, as they all have a low glycemic index (GI). Low GI foods are perfect for endurance, strength and stamina situations, such as labour. Low GI ensures that the blood glucose levels are maintained in a balanced, stable way, releasing the glucose into the bloodstream over a longer period of time. This will provide the body with more energy and stamina for long, established labour situations.

A simple carbohydrate with a high GI can provide a quick hit of glucose into the bloodstream. Perfect examples of these are sugary sports drinks, cordial, lollies or icy poles and chocolate. These suggestions are good for a quick pep-up in energy as the glucose takes next to no time to enter the bloodstream. This is helpful to know in any labour situation, especially if a woman is feeling a little flat. A quick GI fix is ideal in both a fast and a long labour situation, if a woman feels the need for something in her stomach but does not want anything heavy. Women in labour should avoid sucking on lollipops, as this can cause a woman to subconsciously pull up the pelvic-floor muscles, cervix and lower abdominal muscles, thereby defeating the purpose of what the body should be doing, which is letting go and relaxing down through these muscles.

It is a great idea to take your own filtered fresh water to hospital with you, as I find hospital water can taste really terrible in which case you may not drink as much as you should because of the taste.

Women in labour should drink lots of water and eat ice chips. Ice chips are not so bad in taste and are a great idea as they are cold, which helps keep the mouth/body cooler as well as assisting the body to stay hydrated.

Dehydration needs to be avoided as it is not good for a labouring woman or her baby and may result in having to have a drip of saline put into the back of the woman's hand so she can be fed intravenously. This drip, which is fed through a very fine tube, then stays in the hand for the entire labour. It will mean that a woman in labour has to pull and push a pole on wheels with the saline bag hanging from it for the duration of her labour. This disturbs the woman's ability to get into any positions of her choice, as well as being a distraction from her inward focus.

A woman may dehydrate due to not drinking enough fluids, even though she may appear to be drinking all the time. Sweating profusely and/or constantly throughout the labour and peeing all the time does eliminate a large amount of fluid from the body. As well as drinking plain water, sugared water, cordial and sports drinks watered down are ideal in labour, as they tend to assist in hydration because they are directly absorbed. As I have already mentioned they can also give a little pep-up due to the sugar content. Orange juice, or any other citrus type of juice, should be avoided if possible as they tend to be too acidic. On a few occasions I have seen them come straight back up. Vomiting while in labour is a horrible thing and can be avoided by being aware that citrus drinks are not really suitable. If a woman listens to her body she will know what she needs orally during labour.

It is important to note here that for every second drink taken into the mouth the body does a pee out the other end. This is to prevent the bladder from distending above and beyond its capability. Bladder distension is caused when a woman does not regularly pee, so the bladder gets bigger and bigger, till it looks like a small football under the lower part of the abdomen. The reason to avoid this is that the bladder can get so big that it actually prevents the baby's head from moving downwards into the correct position for birthing.

It is easy to avoid an enlarged bladder if women remember and are prompted to pee from time to time throughout their labour. If it becomes impossible to pee because there is either no urge or it feels like there is no urine, a catheter may be inserted into the urethra to drain the bladder of urine. (Remember that it is a woman's choice to have a catheter and it should not be foisted upon her.) Once inserted, the catheter may or may not be taken out, for example, if a woman is going on to have an epidural the catheter stays in.

While we are on the subject of peeing, we may as well discuss the poo side of things and get it all out in the open. It is true that many women during the course of labour feel the need to poo. This can and does occur when a baby's head is coming down the birth canal due to the force and pressure on the rectum. It is quite normal to do a poo at this time and even before this time if a woman feels the need or urge! Remember the information I wrote about on the sphincters of the body. Well, there is really no stopping the urge if it is there. If a woman tries not to poo and lets the muscles of the anus get tighter and tighter the stress caused could create a haemorrhoid, which is a pain in the arse literally (pun totally intended!).

The bottom line is, if a woman in labour has got to do a poo, just do it and don't hold back. If a woman is in a birthing tub a midwife or support person can always just scoop it out of the water. Pooper-scooping at water births or dry births is one of my main jobs as a doula! Sitting on the toilet when a woman has the sensation to do a poo can also be a very comfortable position, and it is there that a woman can be encouraged to take her time, relax and let the imminent poo come out with ease. At the back of the book I have included a very funny birth story in which I caught a poo in my bare hands in the car of all places! Please read and enjoy this story.

As I have said to my antenatal classes on many occasions, in jest, but with more than a grain of truth:

The important thing is that whatever occurs during a woman's labour she should be respected and honoured and, above all, made to feel at ease with the birthing process and all that goes on. When a woman's vagina is totally open she is in the most vulnerable position of her life. Women often describe it as being totally exposed, in every co ceivable way. Therefore, so subtle should be the wiping away of the poo, the touch of the midwife during a VE, or the mopping up of the liquid goozy ((the name I give to the mucus and bloody bits) from the vagina as they fall upon the floor, that the birthing woman does not feel embarrassed. It is all so natural and perfectly normal and not at all shameful – in this way a sense of dignity is in fact maintained. This concept above all else needs to be accepted and understood by a labouring woman, and by all who choose to support her, so they can assist in the best possible way. Respect of the birthing woman gives her true dignity.

When you are in labour and you enter the labour room, you have to leave your dignity at the door and collect it on the way back out. Nothing about giving birth is dignified, however it is also the most normal and natural event a woman can experience. The sooner women realise this the easier it is to get on with labour, stepping aside getting out of your own way, mentally so physically your body can do the job it is designed to do, letting go of wanting to be in control. Remember, the key to giving birth is about surrendering 100%!

Transition – Maximum Opening Of The Body

Transition is like the final chapter of an epic book: it is a welcome stage of labour as the birth is now getting really close. Transition is often easily recognised by support people and midwives, as a change in personality and body language can occur in the woman. The main reason for this change is the release of high levels of oxytocin and adrenalin within the body. Before the onset of transition a woman may appear to be sleepy, deeply relaxed and calm, not wanting to talk or communicate. With the onset of transition a woman can appear wide-eyed, alert and energised in a short space of time.

The body language can be a dead giveaway when a woman is fully dilated. The stance may be with the hands on the hips, pushing the belly out, or if in the tub a woman may kneel in the very centre of the tub, as I did, and not want to be touched. A woman who I attended just started to shake her head from side to side and groan a deep and primal sound. Another woman I attended had piggyback contractions (they are one upon another, with no break between) while in the shower and went up onto the balls of her feet and tiptoes. She calmly stated at the same time, 'I have had enough, when is it going to be over?' Other women have told me to piss off, get stuffed, and even lashed out at me physically and thrown up, which is said to be another indication of a fully dilated cervix. Here is a great example of transition:

Towards the end of the labour that produced her second, and much larger, child, she worked with tireless energy. 'How many more?' she asked me excitedly, as she rested between the contractions. 'It will soon be here,' I replied. 'Why do you ask so anxiously? I hope that you are not too weary.' 'No, no, not that; but this brings back to me so clearly John's arrival; I can hear his cry and see his fat pink body in my hands. I'm longing for that heavenly feeling again; I simply can't describe it to you. It won't be long now, will it?'

Grantly Dick-Read.

Transition can be indicated by many different verbal and physical responses. Some women will quietly place their hands on their hips and state loudly, 'How much longer?' Other women might get very aggressive, swear and scream, 'When is this bloody baby coming out, I can't take any more.'

I did attend one birth where a woman went totally within herself and quietly pushed out her baby without a sound. It truly was the most amazing birth I have ever witnessed. I do know for a fact that more and more of these types of births are occurring in the United States and Australia with the introduction of Hypnosis for labour, which teaches women how to birth calmly and in a very relaxed way.

With the onset of transition the sense of the location of the contractions can change, from deep within the lower abdominal area to the lower back and bottom. It can feel exactly like you have got to do a poo, which in most cases is the baby's head pushing on the coccyx bone, rectum and anus. If there is any poo it will be forced out at this stage, as I have previously mentioned.

However, often women are empty of actual poo and what they perceive as the need to do a poo is in fact the urge to push out the baby! The really good news about this welcoming sensation is that the end of labour is certainly near when a woman feels this pressure from the baby's head. During my first birth I distinctly remember feeling like I had to keep on pooing and pushing and pooing. Looking back I think I felt I was giving birth to poo (others will tell you they gave birth to a small watermelon!). The urge to push never went away, until the top of Jaeosha's head hit my perineum. Then I knew that it was my baby about to be born.

It's important during this stage of labour that the support people give 110 per cent verbal encouragement and support. The power of positive words during this time can assist in not only getting a woman to the fully dilated state, but helping her really believe she can keep on going. When I suggest verbal encouragement, I don't mean yelling or saying to a woman, like a football coach: 'You can do it, you can do it, you can do it!', 'Come on, come on, come on, come on!', or, worse still, 'Push, push, push, push, come on, you can do it!' In fact, many doctors and hospital midwives do use this type of language, without giving the woman time and space to tune into the urge to push by herself, in her own natural timing. An outside person's instructions can be distracting to say the least, but, more importantly, it is another situation where performance anxiety can affect a woman's natural progress and really hinder and interfere with what feels like the right way to go about pushing.

Instead, what I am suggesting is that the words are softly spoken and encouraging:

'Your body is opening up beautifully right now!'
'Visualise your birth canal, completely open like a flower!'

'You are doing a wonderful job of getting your baby down through the birth canal!'

Ina May Gaskin writes about the sphincters of the vaginal area during this transitional stage of labour:

I cannot count how many times I have observed women experiencing similar relaxation of the cervical sphincter that correlated with positive and loving words spoken during the most intense phase of labour (usually around the time the cervix is almost completely open).

It is also really important to let the woman know that she can push her baby out in her own time (unless there is a genuine emergency). Doctors will often rush this stage and use forceps or the suction cap if they believe the woman is not progressing according to hospital protocols. Some hospitals allow only two hours for pushing, but as long as the baby is actually progressing down the birth canal, I believe women should be allowed to take the time they need to work with their body to get their baby out. Again, if rushed, performance anxiety can result, which can totally hinder this natural process by causing the sphincter to be held tight.

Some examples of appropriate words used by a loving partner in labour might be:

'You look so beautiful at this time!'
'I love that you are giving birth to our baby!' 'I love you so much!'
'I think you are doing the most incredible job of birthing our baby.'

All of the above comments help tremendously in assisting a woman to push her baby down through the cervix and into the birth canal. I remember my husband Jerome telling me how wonderful I looked just as I was pushing Jarrad through my cervix. His words at that time made me feel so supported and loved, not to mention strong, and before long I could feel Jarrad was totally through my cervix and on his way down the birth canal ready to be born.

The Dreaded Anterior Lip

Before I continue on this *beautiful birth* journey I feel it is important to explain about the anterior lip, as many women seem to get to transition only to be told not to push as they have an anterior lip. So what is an anterior lip?

An anterior lip occurs when the cervix swells beyond its normal size. The baby will do damage if pushed down and through a swollen cervix, resulting in more swelling, which can prevent the progress of the baby down and through this band of tissue. A woman should never try to push too early in her labour, thinking that this will help the baby down, as it can cause the cervix to swell. Too many vaginal examinations may also be the cause of the soft, tender tissue swelling. A midwife friend of mine also observed a woman in the last stages of labour spending a long time on a fitball, possibly causing an anterior lip, due to perhaps too much force and pressure on the cervix. It is possible that extended periods of fitball sitting, with the legs apart, may cause the pelvis to be so wide that the pressure on the cervix from the baby's head becomes too great, causing it to swell.

If a vaginal examination is done just prior to transition and it is found that a woman has an anterior lip, there are things that she can do to reduce the swelling of the cervix and assist it to get out of the way. Being in the right position is the most important consideration here. If a woman with an anterior lip can get into a horizontal position and reduce the gravitational pull downwards she will be reducing the pressure of the baby's head on the cervix. Therefore, a woman could get onto her elbows and knees with her bottom up in the air and breathe through her contractions for the required period of time. This same position immersed in a big tub of hot water can also reduce the swelling, as the water relaxes the body and the horizontal body-positioning helps reduce the pressure on the cervix.

If a woman is asked to lay on the bed on her back (laying on her side is a better option as the pelvis can still open up) to rest and take the pressure off the cervix, what often happens is that the contractions intensify so greatly that a woman often feels out of control and scared of the contractions as they come. As a result of this heightened intensity in sensation, women may opt for gas to take the edge off the contractions, as well as to assist in focusing on breathing through the contractions. The hardest part about being in this situation is that it is paramount that a woman stays absolutely focused and calm and does not attempt to push at all. She must resist the urge to do so at all costs until given the all clear. Another VE may be necessary to check that the lip has moved out of the way so the pathway down through the cervix into the birth canal is clear.

The Birthing Part Of Labour
– Climbing The Mountain!

The second stage of labour is the most exciting. During the first stage the cervix has thinned out and opened. At the end of the first stage the cervix is open to 10 cm, making the uterus and vagina one birth canal. Then follows a wonderful time when you begin to push. The second stage of labour is often described as if it were sheer, grinding, hard work, but you want to do it. You probably have an overpowering urge to bear down and press the baby through the birth canal. This is passionate, intense, thrilling and often completely irresistible and for some women it is the nearest thing to overwhelming sexual excitement.
Sheila Kitzinger, The New Pregnancy and Childbirth.

The best part of labour, in my opinion, is the pushing part, because all of the contractions you have previously greeted and said goodbye to have been for one purpose and function: to fully dilate the cervix, ready for pushing and moving the baby down into the birth canal to be born. It can feel strangely orgasmic and very satisfying at the same time.

It has been written and documented that this change in sensation from opening to pushing, and movement downwards, can feel like a prolonged sort of orgasmic feeling, which some women find very pleasurable.

In Ina May's Guide to Childbirth, she writes:

Curious about how many women I could find who had orgasmic experiences in labour and birth, I decided to conduct a small survey among some close friends. Of 151 women, I found thirty-two who reported experiencing at least one orgasmic birth. That is twenty-one percent – considerably higher than I had expected.

To back her research Ina May Gaskin goes onto to quote 'Paula' in her book:

I have been pondering this question for some time. I have always felt that labour and birth were like one big orgasm. The contractions were like waves of pleasure rippling through the body. I only found the final few centimeters of dilation as extremely strong and slightly less pleasurable. But I felt like labour and birth were/are a continuous orgasm. I can't say that it is like the orgasm experienced during sexual intercourse, where I find myself being engulfed and lost in a wave of orgasm. The type I experienced during labour and birth was a more all-consuming feeling that required more of my attention than that experienced during sex. However, I do feel that it is an orgasm. The birth itself is very orgasmic as the baby comes through the birth canal – extremely pleasurable and rewarding.

Positioning Is Everything!

One of the best positions to be in for the pushing stage of labour is an upright position (leaning forwards) as gravity can really assist to bring the baby down the birth canal. It goes without say that laying on your back means that a woman is pushing without the assistance of gravity, working against that which nature has kindly provided. As I have already mentioned, Rob Horowitz and Pam England say that there is a significant decrease in the size of the pelvis when lying on the back. This position is not conducive to assisting the pelvis to open and help the baby pass through the pelvic bones, especially if it is a tight squeeze in the first place, such as a normal pelvis and bigger baby.

When a woman is giving birth to a big baby what often happens is that the baby's fontanels (areas between bones of the skull) start to move and shift over each other and mould according to the shape of the mother's pelvis. The bigger the pelvic space the less need for moulding or caput (the slight swelling of the top of a baby's head). Some babies need plenty of time to mould their little fontanels and this is why some second stages of labour take longer than others.

If a woman does push for a considerable amount of time, say for over an hour, she may feel the baby is stuck and not moving. It can be useful to know exactly what is going on internally by tuning in to your body. A change in position may just be what is needed at this stage, to help the baby move down further into the birth canal. If a woman in labour feels she needs more time at this point and the baby's heartbeat is fine, then ask for more time and request that your care providers trust your instinct and remain patient.

I had a woman explain to me how she was given just one hour to push her baby down into her birth canal, and after just one hour she still had no urge to push. The 'need to poo' sensation just never came. She started asking questions of her care provider, who explained, to her dismay, 'The baby is *probably* facing the wrong way, so it could be posterior and is possibly a big baby.' The words this woman clung on to were 'posterior' *'wrong way'* and *'big'*. As she was wheeled up the ramp to the main hospital for an 'epidural' and *'assisted delivery'* she felt defeated in some respects as to why her body had let her down, but was still mentally saying positive affirmations to create some change in the situation. Over and over she was internally repeating to her- self, 'Come on, baby, move down; come on, body, open up'.

Just as she was being prepared for the epidural, she told me how she had the almighty urge to push. And just as 'push came to shove', she didn't tell the staff for fear of ridicule and the fact she had committed herself to having pain relief and had a room full of people waiting to assist her. She felt that if she spoke up at that time it would have been inconvenient for everyone in the room. As a result she had an epidural that lead to a forceps delivery with a rather large episiotomy, which took quite a long time to recover from. Had she spoken out the outcome may have been very different. It is about exercising choice and not being afraid to speak out.

The main point I am trying to make about the above story is that it is never too late to tell your care providers that things have changed. During the course of a labour so many things can change from second to second and minute to minute. That is the wonderful thing about childbirth. It is a true mystery that cannot be controlled by anyone unless you give him or her permission to do so.

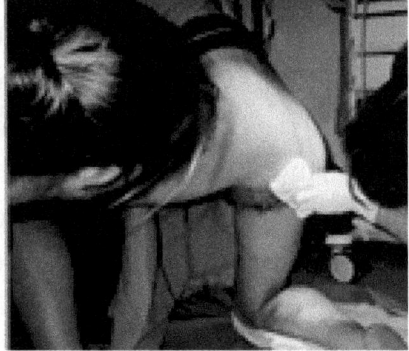

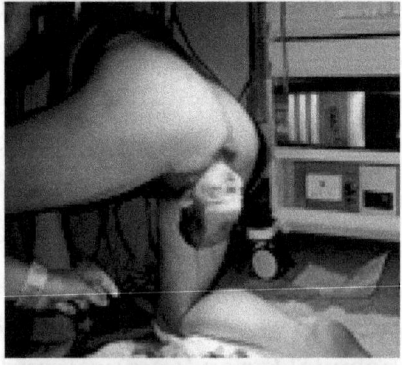

When a baby is coming down the birth canal, positioning is everything and can be the reason some women just stop progressing, as if the cogs of motion have come to a halt. An interesting activity that I learned from one of Australia's childbirth educators, Andrea Robertson, was about pelvic opening and body positioning. Andrea suggests that pregnant

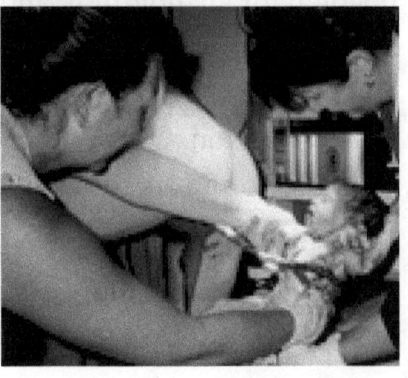

women feel their own pelvis opening by placing one hand on the pubic bone while the other hand is on the tailbone in a squatting or kneeling position. Lean your body back and feel the movement in the pelvis, now lean forward till your torso is nearly parallel to the floor. Most women are surprised to feel just how much further apart their hands felt when they leaned forward. Up to two inches in difference in some cases! Just think how effective those two inches could be if you are birthing a big baby!

Why do care providers ask women to get on the bed?

One of the reasons women are asked to 'pop up on the bed like a good girl' (AARRGGH, I actually heard a midwife request this once) is that a woman's care providers may want to see what is going on. They feel that they can't see if you are down on the floor! One obstetrician told a woman in my class that under no circumstances would he permit her to give birth down on the floor as he had a bad back and it would be too difficult for him to contemplate. Besides, he would not be able to see what was going on! What really is there to see? If the cervix is fully dilated and the baby is well and truly moving down the birth canal the only thing that needs to be observed and controlled is the stretch of the perineum as the head comes through this sensitive tissue.

On a more positive note, I have been at many births where the care provider has got down onto the floor with no hesitation to receive a baby into their waiting hands. On some occasions a torch has been used, just to check on how quickly a baby is descending and only so the care provider could gauge whether to call a doctor or to get the gloves on. The position a woman decides on birthing in is her choice and should not be decided by anyone else. Women need to be aware that the biomechanics of the pelvis and coccyx are designed so that the pelvis can open up and move to its full potential in the forward upright position and not on the back, which causes compression of the pelvic girth.

Women will often ask me, 'If I am in an upright position and I push, won't the baby come out too quickly and tear me?' I usually respond to this question by suggesting that a woman write in her birth plan clearly that she will first and foremost decide and choose the birthing position she feels she would like. And secondly, that she would like her care provider to talk her through the last stage of labour-making suggestions to pant, slow down, or use a keyword like 'back off' or 'gently' to protect her perineum from stretching too quickly and tearing. This type of gentle coaching can help a woman stay upright and birth without tearing. There are many wonderful midwives who will naturally do this anyway as part of their service and care.

From my experience, the urge to just push and get the baby out is so overwhelming that women often do just push as hard as they possibly can. Women are putting themselves in a situation where they could sustain a tear if they do push uncontrollably. Therefore, it is imperative that a woman highlights in her birth plan that she be talked and coached through the pushing stage by whoever is present in the room. This is not necessarily something a woman will remember to ask her caregivers when she is at this point of labour, due to the intensity and focus needed. It is more helpful if her support person points to the birth plan, where this point is strongly highlighted, or have her support person ask that this request be actualised.

At this point of labour, panting through the mouth can also assist in slowing down the need to push, as it does take the focus off bearing down. It is important to note that inhalation should be strong and direct so hyperventilation and dizziness does not result. It is potentially very dangerous to hold the breath while bearing down with all your force and strength. This is known as a 'Valsalva manoeuvre' and can result in the capillaries in the whites of the eyes bursting, as well as the blood pressure sky-rocketing up into dangerous highs, not to mention causing hemorrhoids. Damage may also be caused to the pelvic-floor muscles as they are pushed and stretched with great force.

Elizabeth Noble in her book Childbirth With Insight, writes:

A considerable amount of blood pools in the pelvis during the Valsalva Manoeuver, because the blood cannot return to the heart against the high pressure in the chest. The veins which in pregnancy are dilated more easily due to hormonal softening, are thus predisposed to varicosities such as hemorrhoids.

I witnessed a midwife gently placing her hand on the baby's head as it was coming through the perineum to slow the movement down, as she asked the woman to pant through her mouth. To my amazement the perineum retracted back and over the baby's head to the neck, while the woman had no contraction occurring at this time. The body just gently stretched and expelled the baby of its own accord. When the next contraction did finally arrive, the body of the baby just slid gently out into my hands. It was so peaceful and calm, and without a tear or a graze to the perineum.

Another birth I attended was for a friend who had sustained a very big tear during the birth of her first baby. She had decided to have me assist her as a doula, to look after her perineum, among other things! When we arrived at the birthing centre, she instinctively took up a position on the floor, lying on her side with her head under the double bed, with just her body exposed.

It was here that I relayed to her to 'back off', 'pant', 'back off', 'pant', etc. At this point she could only identify with my voice, and did as she was instructed beautifully and birthed with one leg in the air on her side, as her very big baby boy came into the world, without a tear to mum's perineum. The lying-on-the-side position is ideal for women who really need to slow down the pushing stage of labour to avoid a tear.

It is really unnecessary for a care provider to run their finger around the perineum as used to be done, as this can further stretch the perineal tissue beyond its capacity, actually causing the perineum to split and tear further. The soft tissue of the perineum is best left alone during the maximum stretch of birth. The next chapter highlights how the best perineal preparation can be achieved, which is during the weeks leading up to the birthday.

22

How To Prepare The Perineum

The perineum is a wonderful part of the female anatomy, as not only does it open like a flower, but it grows in size and shape to gently pass over a baby, from the tip of a baby's head all the way to the toes. Without this wonderful tissue a baby's entrance into the world would probably be one of shock, as the baby would fly out of the body and not enter in the calm, massaged and gentle way that it does.

Some women stretch and open beautifully with no tearing of the perineum. During my births I sustained no tearing at all, just grazes inside. This is probably due to my waterbirths, as most women that water-birth very rarely tear; it is thought that the warm water, added salt and relaxation qualities of the water assist the perineum to give and stretch. Therefore no tearing occurs.

However, there are exercises that can be done to assist the perineum to stretch. Stretching the perineum in the lead-up to the birth can really help it to give during the maximum stretch required when the baby's head emerges. Many women that I have supported over the years swear by the benefits gained by practising 'perineal massage'.

Perineal massage not only improves the stretch and give of this tissue, but also improves the circulation of blood, relaxation of the tissue and, most importantly, the elasticity. When warm, cold-pressed olive oil, or apricot oil, is used in conjunction with the massage the result can be a softer, more flexible perineum.

Perineal massage could be started about four to six weeks before a woman's estimated date, with the massage taking up five minutes every few days. It can be awkward but not impossible for women to actually do the stretches and massage themselves, so to make this easier it is a good idea to have your partner do it for you. I did have a friend who was actually determined to do this stretching herself. With one leg up on the chair, oil on the fingers and thumbs, and with a mirror on the floor, she set about to open, release and stretch her perineum. Pulling with the hand/fingers at the front and the other hand/fingers from behind she stretched her own perineum tissue apart.

She was doing PNF stretching. PNF stands for Proprioceptive Neuromuscular Facilitation. Which basically means you stretch as far as you can go, holding the stretch for about six to ten seconds, then you let go and have a rest. You then stretch again, going a little further and holding for six to ten seconds, and repeat a third and final time. In this case my friend went as far as she could without causing herself any unnecessary stress or strain, but just a little sensation of discomfort, and all the while she focused on her labour breathing technique. As a result of doing this kind of stretch (and as I witnessed at the birth as her doula) she felt very little burning or stinging when the perineum was bulging as her baby's head came through and sustained no tear or graze.

Partner perineal massage is a lot easier because a woman can relax her body, while her partner is doing the necessary stretches. This also enables a woman to focus on her breath and work through any discomfort and sensations that are being experienced, all of which is great preparation for the actual crowning of the baby's head on the birth-day.

The best position for a woman to be in is semi-reclined, lying back on pillows, with her legs bent up and slightly opened. A woman's partner, with warm oil on his thumbs and fingers, slides his thumbs into the vagina, applying pressure down towards the anus first, slowly pressing down and outwards, making the letter U with the thumbs just inside the vagina. The pressure needs to be firm and strong, however not unbearable. A pregnant woman will need to communicate to her partner whether the pressure is adequate or not, so make sure that the talking continues throughout this exercise. This U-shape pressure stretch can be repeated two or three times depending on how a woman feels at that moment.

Protecting The Perineum During The Birth

Despite all this preparation, care still needs to be taken so that this tissue does not tear during the crowning of the baby's head. As I have already mentioned, when the time comes to push the baby out of the body there is an overwhelming urge to push, especially when a woman starts to feel the 'Ring of Fire' or 'Chinese Burn'. So strong is this feeling that women forget what they are doing and just push anyway, to rid themselves of this burning, stinging feeling. (Or with some women, the urge to push is so overwhelming that they push hard and fast without even stopping to think.)

Staying focused and aware of not pushing fast and hard is the key. My suggestion is to have a woman who is in labour frequently apply by hand a plain, cold-pressed apricot oil to her perineum and surrounding tissue to help it stay soft and supple. This is especially important if the woman has been getting in and out of the shower and tub, as the skin does tend to dry out, even though there are natural goozys slowly descending from the birth canal that do assist with lubrication.

Hot compresses on the perineum can be very effective in taking the sting out of the stretching tissue. I have used hot compresses at many births and women always comment on just how fantastic it is to feel the heat from the cloth instantly. The only problem with having hot cloths available and ready is finding a spare pair of hands to get a container suitable, the cloths ready and the water hot enough to make a difference. This is relatively easy at home. However, most hot water that comes out of the taps in hospitals would not be hot enough to provide any form of relief. A support person would need to find out where the kitchen is and use boiled water from the urn or kettle with a dash of cold. A way of testing the temperature of the water before applying the cloth to a woman's perineum is to place a cloth on your forearm for a moment. If you can leave it there comfortably for a period of time without it burning, it is suitable for the perineum. As a support person, always test the cloth on your forearm first. It should be hot but not burning!

Avoiding an episiotomy

If perineal massage has been practised during the weeks leading up to the start of labour and a woman has no fear surrounding the pushing stage of birth, she has done all that she can to prevent a tear, and the likelihood of her having or needing an episiotomy is very remote. However, if the time comes and the soft tissue of her perineum needs to give a little more she could be faced with the prospect of either tearing or being cut. The choice is one which will need to be made in the moment. Some obstetricians will automatically perform an episiotomy (cut of the perineal skin) with little to no thought for a woman's well-being and recovery, while other obstetricians and midwives will let a woman tear, as they feel this heals better.

Sheila Kitzinger, in her book The New Pregnancy and Childbirth, writes about problems associated with episiotomy:

A trial conducted in Dublin revealed that women with an intact perineum or only superficial tear experience less pain after childbirth than those who have an episiotomy. The pain after an episiotomy is about the same as that from a second degree tear (one that affects the underlying muscle). Women are more likely to have severe tears into the anus when they have had an episiotomy, than if they had not had one. Another trial in England showed that there is no advantage in episiotomy over a first or second degree tear.

Someone once told me a great analogy that really represents the whole concept of an episiotomy, and that is: If you were to pick up a piece of material and try to tear it with your own bare hands the material will resist tearing. But, if you were to cut this material just a little bit first with a pair of scissors it would show little resistance when tension was applied and a tear would occur all the way till the pressure stopped. This analogy can apply to the perineum tissue as well.

Included in *Ina May's Guide to Childbirth*, is evidence to suggest that having an episiotomy is like a female version of genital mutilation. Interestingly enough, according to Ina May, all claims that are said to be for the benefit of helping a woman and her baby in their time of need have been found to be:

> *...without any supporting evidence by doctors or hospitals all over North America. An episiotomy is supposed to assist in preventing urinary and fecal incontinence, save the baby from shoulder dystocia (where the baby's shoulders get stuck), and make the job of sewing up afterwards easier, prevent the baby from being oxygen deprived, preventing brain damage and mental retardation!*

Ina May also goes on to write that:

> *... plenty of research has since been done and the findings have supported that which many a midwife and woman has suspected all along. That is, a routine episiotomy has no benefit and carries many serious disadvantages.*

Ina May summarises the possible problems with episiotomies, that they:

- Cause pain that sometimes lasts for weeks or months.
- Increase blood loss.
- Cause more serious tears because a cut perineum is not as resistant to lacerations as an intact one.
- Often become infected.
- Are associated with wound breakdown, abscesses, permanent damage to the pelvic-floor muscles, and other complications that do cause incontinence.
- Prevent women from breastfeeding in a seated position

because of the pain they feel caused from the stitches they have.

- Make sitting and walking sometimes unbearable, especially if the stitches are very tight and there are a lot of them.

To conclude, therefore, I suggest that a little stretching and attention given to perineal massage during the weeks leading up to the birth-day can prevent one aspect of tissue trauma that really could be avoided. Like many suggestions in this book, it is about choice and a woman's right to choose what she does and does not do to prepare herself.

23
The Arrival of Your Cherub

One of the greatest moments of birth is undoubtedly the arrival of your baby into your arms. In an instant the sweat and hard work are all but forgotten, and the world seems to stand still for a while, as you contentedly look into your baby's eyes for the very first time.

This is the moment women long for and work towards tirelessly, contraction after contraction. This is the top of the mountain, when you have reached the summit. This is a moment that can never be repeated or felt again physically, but in memory only. Words are hard to find to describe the first moment of being skin to skin with your baby for the very first time. Only a mother with this memory will appreciate my enthusiasm for the experience. This moment above all others should be honoured and treasured as it can come and go so very quickly.

No woman ever forgets the first screams of her baby – it demands so much, it is vehement and appealing and yet the infant is so helpless of itself to survive. It is a call that vitalises mother love and the maternal sense awakens to protect, comfort, and care for the child.

When a baby finally arrives and comes into the world on that last big contraction, the feeling of sheer relief and ecstasy are entwined. For most women there is disbelief that something so beautiful and perfect could have grown and come from within them. I remember at the birth of my daughter, Jaeosha, how I kept repeating to myself, 'Oh my God, it is a baby!' I don't know whether I thought it was going to be some kind of alien creature or something. All I knew was that I could not believe that I had just given birth to a baby. Many births I have attended have ended with the exact words I used myself: 'Look, it is a baby.' I think that women get so caught up in the whole labour experience that they forget that the finale of this epic journey is the pot of gold at the end of the rainbow.

Birthing a baby is the most wonderful part of labour. Women should not fear this stage, as the birthing of a baby through the birth canal is truly a miracle. For a brief moment in time a baby is between the two worlds of life, ready to leave one behind and begin the new. It is a time for a woman to accept her graduation from the life she has previously known and lived to a totally new experience. Things are never going to be the same again.

When a baby is born, it is important to have the baby placed on the mother's chest, skin to skin. The skin-to-skin contact is important for a few reasons. Firstly, it keeps the baby warm, and secondly, it provides the baby with an opportunity to smell their mother and feel close. This time together ensures bonding between mother and baby and also assists in the production of oxytocin in the mother. Oxytocin (the love hormone) is produced

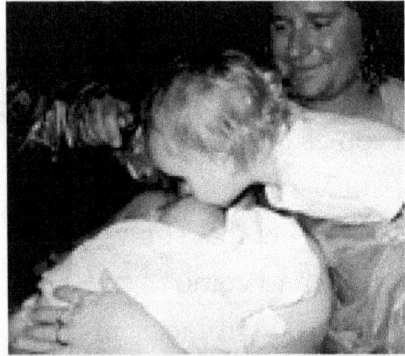
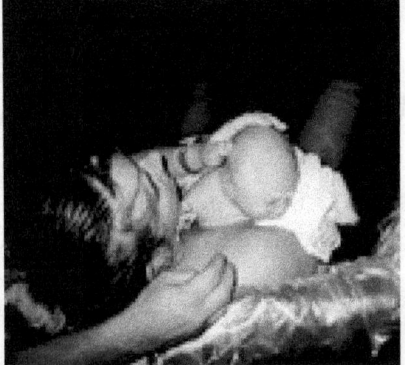
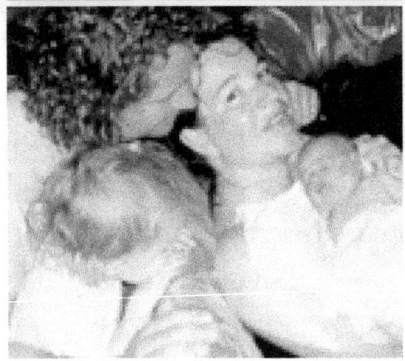

in the mother when cuddling her baby and it is heightened by the skin-to-skin contact. This assists the 'falling in love with the baby' process. The production of oxytocin also aids in the release of the placenta and preparation for breastfeeding the baby.

Birth represents a new beginning, a new journey, and prepares women for the everyday hardships of being a parent and mother. The challenge and intensity of birth assists a woman to feel strong and confident about her role as a mother and strengthens the bond that she has with her baby. After a period of time and the birthing of a baby, things in life alter, change and seem different – previously important issues less important. Priorities tend to change, as does one's attitude towards things that perhaps were considered very important before the baby was born. All of these changes are necessary and totally normal; they are essential to ensure that a mother's priority is her baby, that nothing else matters. Take the time to enjoy your baby, as you can never turn back the clock and have this moment or day again.

Birthing The Placenta

The good news about birthing the placenta is that it feels like a big, soft jellyfish.

The third stage of labour is very much a case of leaving the easy part till last. Although contractions are still present for a lot of women after the birth of the baby, they feel toned down in intensity and are often quite comfortable to bear. The afterbirth contractions are necessary to assist the placenta in detaching from the wall of the uterus.

There are two ways in which women can expel their placenta, and that is with or without synthetic syntometrine being administered through a needle in the thigh. When syntometrine is not used it is known as a physiological third stage, in which the placenta is expelled in its own time. This is an option for women and their partners to consider. However, having said that, one of the reasons that syntometrine may be necessary is in a situation where a woman is bleeding quite heavily. The syntometrine works by shutting down the capillaries of the uterus, hence causing a quick explosion (shuffling off) of the placenta from the wall of the uterus. The blood loss then slows down and a woman is considered to be bleeding in a controlled, normal manner.

In many hospitals there always seems to be a big rush to get the placenta out. Waiting, rather than rushing, allows the last of the placental and cord blood to flow into the baby and allows the cord to stop pulsating. The benefit of this is that the baby continues to receive the mother's hormones and red blood cells, which help to give the baby a good start in health.

Hospitals, on the other hand, tend to favour cord clamping at the first opportunity. Those who are critical of the assembly-line approach point out that pre-empting the physiological process is likely to increase problems such as retained placenta, postpartum hemorrhage, and respiratory distress in babies. Studies have shown that delayed cord clamping allows between twenty and fifty percent of the baby's blood volume to flow into the baby. Early cord clamping also results in lower hematocrit or hemoglobin values in the newborn (fewer red blood cells).

To check and see if the cord has stopped pulsating, all you have to do is hold it in your hand and feel if there is a pulse of blood moving through the cord. If there is, ask for more time as you believe the cord is still pulsating. It is really great if your partner can cut the cord (if they are not too queasy), but do warn them, it is like a tough rope to cut and requires some effort. Alternatively, a sibling who has been present at the birth may like to cut the cord.

Sometimes a placenta takes a longer time to expel from the body during a physiological third stage than during a drug-assisted third stage. Having the baby suck on the breast can assist the uterus to continue contracting, which in turn will aid in the expulsion of the placenta naturally. (Immediate breastfeeding and sucking of nipples/breast also helps with bonding and connection between mother and baby, which certainly assists in establishing good breastfeeding from the outset of the birth.)

Putting a baby to the breast elicits a flow of two hormones – oxytocin and prolactin which work together to stimulate milk production. Oxytocin causes muscle contraction and plays an important function in breastfeeding, as it squeezes muscles in the milk ducts and leads to milk ejection. It also makes the uterus contract, so breastfeeding soon after birth helps the uterus tighten and prevents haemorrhage.

What Could I Do With The Placenta?

You do have a choice to keep your placenta or to leave it behind in the hospital. If you decide to take it home there are two things that you can do with it. Firstly you can plant it under a fruit tree or plant, preferably not under Australian native trees as it will kill them. The other alternative is to eat a small portion of your placenta. This is known as placentophagy. I can hear the majority of you now saying, 'Oh that is disgusting, gross, foul', etc., etc. I thought that at first as well, but having eaten a small portion of two placentas I can honestly say it made a huge difference to how I felt and coped during my postpartum period.

Like many women who have just given birth to a baby, I felt a little teary and emotional. It is really not unusual for women who have just given birth to feel unsettled and a little down during the days that follow the birth of their baby. It does not necessarily mean that you are suffering from postnatal depression, but simply that you are adjusting to a major life change that goes way beyond the physical changes of the body. Sleep deprivation can play a huge part in feeling down and depressed, not to mention the ongoing demands of breastfeeding.

I certainly wasn't expecting that I was going to be a little depressed, teary and emotional. So on day three, when my milk came in just after the birth of my first baby, Jaeosha, I was all of those things, and eating the placenta seemed like the best thing to do at the time. Immediately I noticed a difference in the way I felt on various levels, emotionally, mentally and physically, and I seemed to have more energy to cope with my life changes.

I really never thought I would be one of those people to attempt something so uncommon as eating my own placenta. However, when the time came there was no real question of whether or not I would, I just felt compelled to do so. Admittedly, I was very interested and amazed at what a placenta looked like and had my midwife show me in absolute detail what it was all about, especially the first time I birthed this amazing thing that my body had created. The thought of eating some just didn't faze me at all. In hindsight, I think that you have to feel attracted to your placenta in order to eat any. If it looks calcified and grainy it is not attractive, hence you won't feel like having any. I believe that if you have this attraction it indicates that the placenta obviously has something in it that your body needs to give you a lift and a pick-me-up. The reason I suggest this is that with the birth of my second baby, Benjamin, I didn't feel at all attracted to his placenta, and as a consequence didn't feel like I needed to have any at all.

Midwife Mary Field, RGN, SCM, wrote a paper on her personal experience of this 'unmentionable' practice in November 1984, explaining how after the birth of her first child she suffered terrible depression for months. She goes on to state:

... by the first postpartum day I noticed how old my body had become and how postnatal depression then set in with a vengeance – uncontrollable weeping for hours and, after the first couple of days, I was psychotic.

She describes how her skin felt very dry and coarse and her hair fell out. She felt overwhelmed with emotion and very depressed, even though her birth experience had been pretty straightforward.

Leading up to her second birth Mary was determined to examine ways in which to avoid the same scenario occurring. Mary read the work of Dr Odent and others and knew having a natural childbirth would, to a degree, protect her against most symptoms, but not all. On conclusion of her research and investigation into the benefits of eating the placenta, Mary wrote the following, which I absolutely agree with:

Some types of post natal depression are certainly due to hormone imbalance and readjustment following the birth of the baby – some women readjust well, others, like myself, do not. I decided I not only wanted a natural childbirth, but to try to protect myself from hormone imbalance. The placenta produces and contains female hormones and maintains a high level in the blood during pregnancy; after delivery the hormone level drops down suddenly and the body has to readjust. My theory was that if I ate this tissue, female hormones, which are types of steroids, would be absorbed and make the blood level drop more gradually.

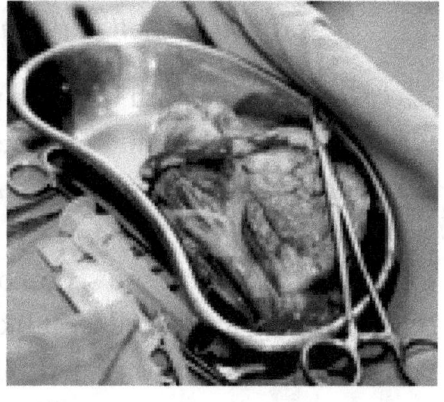

Mary Field, RGN, SCM, 'Placentophagy'.

After the birth of her second child, Mary decided to eat portions of her placenta and proceeded to experiment with ways to ingest the placenta tissue. She tried to fry pieces, which she found to be horrible. Mary then ate some small pieces raw and also knew that making a stew could be a suitable alternative, as the steroids present would not be destroyed if temperatures didn't exceed 100 °C.

The results of eating bits of placenta raw over the next few days after childbirth were described as follows in Mary's own words:

Over the next few days I noticed the physiological effects of my experiment.

The best results were seen in my skin and hair. I retained the bloom of pregnancy over the first postpartum week and even the skin of my belly seemed supple, not dry as with Sarah, my first child, while my hair was silky and shining. I remembered that human placentae used to be sent to some cosmetic firms to make extracts for beauty care. My milk supply was abundant by the second day. Postnatal euphoria set in – I was so strong and felt as though I could do anything.

Like Mary, I found the best way to eat portions of placenta was to have very small amounts of placenta cut up into pieces that were then frozen on a tray. A plastic ice-cube tray is perfect as you can put one piece in each square on the tray so they don't touch. This way you can scoop out a piece, placing it at the back of your throat, and swallow it like a tablet with water. If you find you can still taste it you can dip it in yoghurt first, then swallow with water. It really is just like taking a tablet if you make the pieces small enough. The key to cutting up the placenta into nice small amounts is cutting it up immediately while it is fresh and not frozen. The large part of the placenta that you don't cut up can then be frozen as a back-up if more is required later on. If this part of the placenta is not consumed it can then be planted under a tree and you could have a ceremony and celebration, a dedication to your baby.

Like Mary, I too felt really uplifted, content and calm after eating the placenta over a period of about four to five days. This was just long enough for my milk to come in, the afterbirth pains to subside, not to mention the heavy, sore vaginal feeling to dissipate. Life was looking up, and the feeling that Mary described as 'postnatal euphoria' was abundantly present when I ate the placenta. I speak from experience of having eaten placenta after two births out of three, and from this I concluded that overall I did feel very different and more able to cope with having a new-born baby when I ate portions of the placenta, compared to not having it.

With the epidemic of postnatal depression prevalent in western society, it is a shame to rule out the possibility that the placenta may hold some important hormones that the body needs in order to cope with this type of depression. I know there are huge psychological barriers surrounding the practice of placentophagy, but what if this is the missing recipe for prevention right under our noses? Surely the thought of eating one's own placenta is not that outrageous and abhorrent that a woman would avoid doing so and suffer unnecessarily in the throes of despair and depression?

This practice is about choice, but I want to ask of the women reading this book not to dismiss this idea based on what others might think. Besides, you don't have to tell anyone you want to or are eating portions of your placenta.

24

Breastfeeding – The Nectar From The Gods

The breast is best!

I am including this chapter on breastfeeding as it is an obvious follow-on from birthing your baby, especially if you are planning to put your baby to your breast when he/she is born.

Although I consider myself quite well-informed about breastfeeding, having fed three children for two years each, I should mention that I am not a lactation consultant. If you want to prepare for breastfeeding during your pregnancy, then I suggest you choose a book from your local women's health centre. And if you do need help breastfeeding your new baby, don't hesitate to get urgent help from a lactation consultant. Some lactation consultants work at the maternity hospitals and others practise independently. It is a good idea to have the phone number of a lactation consultant handy on the fridge door so that if you need help you can quickly and easily make a call.

A question that I often get asked about breastfeeding is, 'How will I be able to breastfeed if I have not had prior leakage of colostrum while pregnant?' Women often assume because they have not had any signs of their breasts leaking that they are empty. However, this is not the case at all. I myself was very surprised when my breasts showed no colostrum at all prior to having my first baby, but this did not affect in any way the amount of milk that I was able to produce after the birth. If anything, I could have been a wonderful wet nurse, supplying a whole neighbourhood of babies with breast milk!

From my experience, breastfeeding for approximately six years, I found it to be both challenging and a wonderful experience. In fact, the day I decided to wean my third child was a very sad day for me. I really didn't want to stop feeding my little cherub. What I really loved about breastfeeding is the fact that your milk is on tap, which requires no preparation at all. Secondly, the one-on-one contact and nurturing experienced by both mother and baby is wonderful and enables a close bonding to take place. I loved nothing more than my babies rolling back their eyes in sheer ecstasy as my milk flowed freely into their mouth. They looked as if they were in heaven; as they fed from me they would drift off to a place far away.

Breastfeeding is one of those things that even after six years I still considered myself to be a novice at when it was all over with. This is because with every baby I birthed, the breastfeeding that followed seemed to be a new learning experience, when I almost had to start from scratch as to what to do and how to do it. This is because the baby is an important – and very individual – part of the breastfeeding duo.

I really only had one or two months' break in between weaning one toddler in preparation for the next baby. The reason I chose to do that was so I had a break before birthing the next baby and starting breastfeeding with the newborn. Each and every time I had to learn how to attach this new little mouth onto my breast, only to find my nipples would crack and blister and I would sometimes be in severe agony, despite the fact that the attachment was fine according to the lactation consultant.

I came up with my own theory as to why some women, like myself, find breastfeeding painful initially, even though the attachment appears to be fine. From my experience of working alongside lots of women, it is not uncommon for them to experience a little discomfort and pain as a result of breastfeeding for the very first time. Perhaps some women have very tender and sensitive nipples that feel the strain and stress when sucked into the back of a baby's mouth. Oh boy, can a little baby suck hard and really change the shape of a nipple and breast!

Nevertheless, attachment to the breast may be to blame if there are difficulties, and some women do suffer from severe cracks, blisters and bleeding as they get breastfeeding established. I would like to stress that this scenario does not happen to every woman, but it helps to know that breastfeeding may not be straightforward and easy, as it is a learned art and one that our culture does not seem to effectively pass on to our younger women.

For some people breastfeeding really is a simple, no-pain experience right from the first moment, which is wonderful. However, I try to advise women that if they have problems, they should not think they are a failure and get depressed about it. Breastfeeding really is like fitting two pieces of a puzzle together, with one piece big while the other piece is little. It can take work to get the two pieces to fit each other initially, but once the pieces fit, the hard work is over and it is just a matter of going with the flow…

I believe one of the problems with breastfeeding today is that women will quite often see other women out breastfeeding while having a coffee or a conversation with a friend in the park, almost oblivious to the fact she is breastfeeding her baby. To an observer it may appear that breastfeeding is a piece of cake, so when the time comes for a woman to breastfeed her baby and it does not occur smoothly, she may feel a certain degree of stress and incompetence. What the onlooker may not know is that the mother she observed feeding her baby with ease may also have been through some initial discomfort when she first started to breastfeed; she is now over that period and finding it easy (once the baby is around two months old). It is really worth persevering through the first six to eight weeks to establish comfortable breastfeeding.

There are some factors that may contribute to breastfeeding being hard work and I feel it is important to highlight these. Firstly, inverted nipples. These can be pulled out with a 'nipple puller'. A nipple puller is a little bulb that sucks the nipple out, then a woman attaches her baby quickly to keep the nipple from inverting again. Another solution to this problem is to use nipple shields, which fit over the top of a nipple and assist the baby to attach without causing pain or trauma to

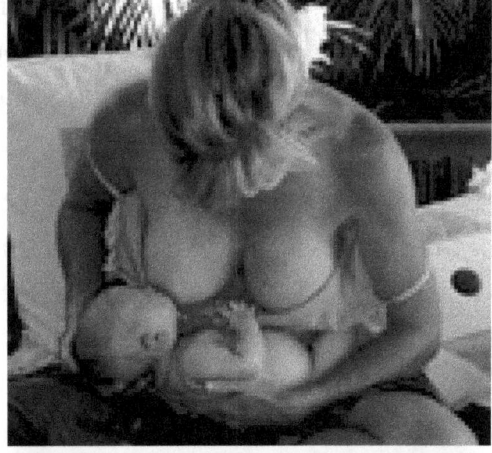
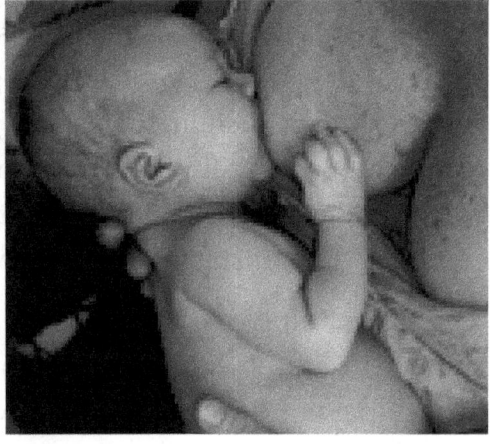

the breast tissue. These are a great alternative for women who are feeling discomfort when feeding. They do, however, take a little getting used to for both mother and baby, and can reduce the hormones produced as a result of breastfeeding.

Secondly, 'latch on' or attachment. When a baby is first born the initial breastfeed is sometimes performed with poor attachment. This may be because assistance is not available, or the new mum may not be sure about correct attachment, hence the baby sucks on just the nipple, causing it to crack and split during this very first attempt to feed.

Babies have an automatic reflex to breastfeed. Good positioning, which supports the baby's head and shoulders close to the breast, will enable the baby's rooting reflex to find the nipple and latch on deeply. The baby should always take into his or her mouth your whole areola, which is the dark pink/brown part of your nipple.

Sometimes the first feed at night can contribute to problems. If the woman is really tired, has a dim light on and gets the baby attached in a way that is not correct, this can contribute to sore nipples and poor milk flow. Allowing your baby to fall asleep on the breast and then taking them off your nipple can cause the nipples to stretch and crack.

The best rule of breastfeeding is that if it hurts or does not feel right to you, stick your little finger into your baby's mouth and break their suction, then start again. By doing this you can eliminate further pain and stress to your nipples. However, if you continue to have pain after re-latching it may be wise to seek out a lactation consultant to really check over what's happening.

Cracked nipples can heal if you allow them some time out and get air onto them. Walking around with nothing covering them or laying down on the bed with a towel to soak up the milk are ideal ways to assist your nipples to heal. Or you could use a hairdryer on a warm setting after each feed. Expressing a little milk and allowing it to dry on your breasts can act like a natural antibiotic. Calendula cream, vitamin E, purified lanolin and natural aloe vera from the plant can be used on the nipples, but do be aware that you will need to wash your nipples before giving your baby a feed. The taste of these creams could put a baby off breastfeeding, especially natural aloe vera direct from the plant. It is really horrible to taste.

If a baby has come through a drug-induced birth experience they may be very tired and sleepy. This is particularly true if pethidine has been used as a form of pain relief. If a baby is like this it maybe incredibly hard for him or her to be interested in breastfeeding, or once you get them latched on they may fall asleep almost immediately. Breastfeeding problems can and do arise from this type of scenario. Giving a baby who is sleepy a bath to wake them up can help, as well as taking off their clothes so they feel a little cool. Perseverance is definitely the key word here. It may take up to a week for a baby to wake up and want to feed.

The ideal time to put your baby on the breast is within the first hour after birth. It is an important part of the way in which you welcome your baby into life and start to get to know each other. The baby's sucking reflex is especially strong during that first hour. If this time is missed, a baby often loses all desire to suck for the next twenty-four hours, seems completely clueless when you try to put her to the breast, or may fuss and fume as if you were trying to force on her something particularly unpleasant.

Sometimes when a mother's milk comes in (around day three to five), engorgement, the swelling of the breast tissue, can make it extremely hard for the baby to attach as the breasts are so enlarged and painful, not to mention hot. Attachment for the baby can be assisted by expressing some milk off the breast before attempting to attach your baby. This can be done with a breast pump or by hand-expressing in the shower, as the heat enables the ducts to open and the milk to flow more easily. Engorgement can also occur if your baby sleeps for long periods of time in between feeds, in which case your milk supply will be abundant. The problem with engorgement is that it can lead to mastitis, which is caused from congestion of the milk ducts and inflammation of the breast tissue.

When breasts are engorged, putting frozen cabbage leaves around the breast tissue helps to soften the tissue and keeps the breast cooler, especially if the leaves are frozen. How do the cabbage leaves work? It sounds so much like an old wives' tale and yet it is a genuine remedy! They release a chemical which penetrates into the skin, which assists the breast tissue to feel soft and supple. If frozen cabbage leaves are used then often within ten minutes the cabbage will be cooked and the aroma of cooked cabbage will emanate from your cleavage. This is a small price to pay for such a wonderful alleviation of discomfort! I answered the door once to the mailman in this strange predicament, having cabbage leaves poking out the top of my maternity bra. It wasn't till after I closed the door that I realised what he was looking at in bemusement. He must have thought I had gone a bit loopy in my postpartum state!

Mastitis is inflammation of the breast tissue in which the breast may feel very hot. There may be red patches on the skin where the ducts are blocked. The thing to really watch out for is a very quick onset of fever, tired, aching muscles and the feeling of coming down with the flu. I distinctly remember sitting in bed feeling sore and engorged in the left breast one minute, then shivering, sweating and shaking the next. I had not expected the onset of this sudden fever to occur so quickly.

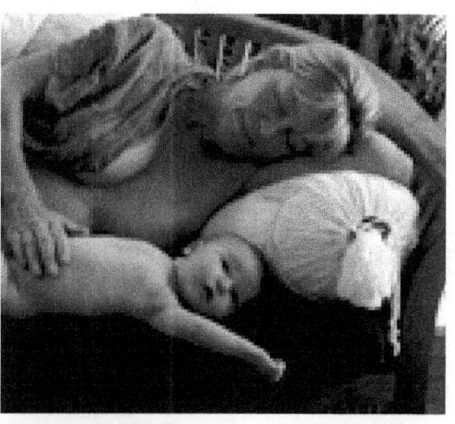

I was very fortunate that I had my midwife at home doing a routine postnatal check when this occurred. How we treated this bout of mastitis was with homeopathics, hand-expressing in the bath, followed by feeding the baby off the sore breast, with correct attachment to get the milk moving through the blocked ducts. Following all of this

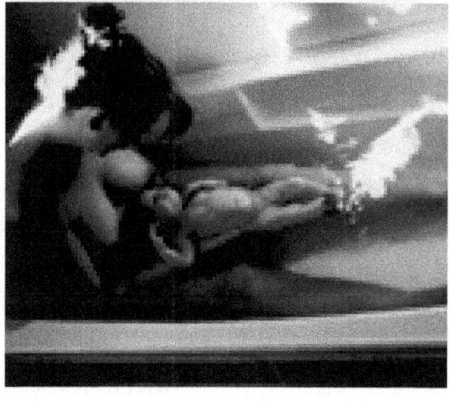

was a trip to the physiotherapist clinic to have some ultrasound treatment on the breast/blocked ducts. From my experience the ultrasound was really fantastic in speeding up the recovery of the blocked duct. Ultrasound can also be used on hemorrhoids and perineal tears to reduce the swelling and enable the tissue to heal .

In order to prevent mastitis, women should try to avoid wearing underwire bras or bras that are too tight. Holding your elbows against your breast tissue when feeding could also cause a blockage. Feeding while lying on your side in bed when your breast is being squashed and flattened can contribute to blocked ducts and mastitis, although feeding lying down is also a great timesaver and well worth figuring out – just don't squash your breasts. The most important thing when faced with the onset of mastitis is to keep feeding your baby off that breast in various positions if you need to, such as the football hold, over the shoulder and in a reversed horizontal position. This can help greatly with emptying the ducts. The red marks on the skin usually indicate where the ducts are blocked.

Getting Enough Sleep

Women have often commented to me about the fact that they love being a mother, they love the breastfeeding, but they find the sleep deprivation the hardest thing to deal with. They are not alone in this. I too found the night feeds very hard to deal with first time around with my daughter. I will say it does get a little easier the more children you have. It is as if your body actually gets used to the disruption and in a strange sort of way you adapt to not having eight hours' sleep per night.

One thing that I always try to encourage first-time mothers to do is sleep when your baby sleeps. This way at least you are getting some rest so the night-time shift does not seem so hard and demanding. To run around cleaning the house when the baby sleeps can be a waste of valuable time when you could be catching up on much-needed sleep, not only for your sake but for the sake of everyone else in the household. Admittedly, it can seem impossible to sleep when everything appears to be such a mess and you have toddlers and other children in the house. This is

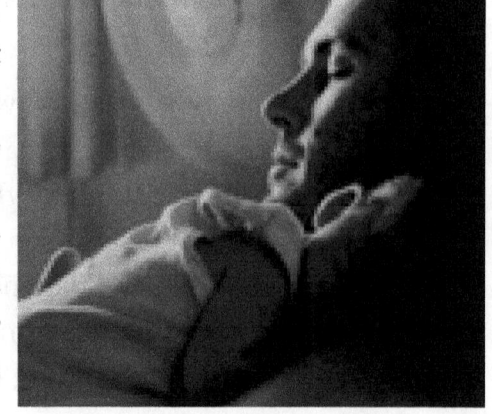

when family and friends can be of great assistance to help a new mum through the initial stage of sleep deprivation by coming around to help out.

The Family Bed

Another way to gain a little more sleep during the night is to have the baby in the bed with you. I had all my babies in my bed up until they were eight months old. After the eighth month I felt it was time to have my bed back and my own space, so my babies went into a cot, but I know many other families sleep with their children for longer than that.

The 'family bed' was a wonderful way to help my baby feel safe and close to me and my husband during the night. It also enabled me to feel close to the baby as I could touch them, smell them and feel them breathing. I could feed lying down so my body stayed relaxed throughout the night. I feel this helped my babies to stay sleepy even though they were breastfeeding. They very rarely cried at night for a feed as all they needed to do was wake up and move their little arms and legs around a little. I always awoke immediately and gave them a feed. I remember one night it felt like my baby was tapping me on the arm, as if to say, 'Come on, Mum, get your breast out, it's feed time.' Once the breastfeed was over we all drifted off to sleep together. It was a very calm and wonderful experience having them right next to me for those eight months.

A lot of people don't advocate the family bed because of the risk of rolling on the baby or smothering the baby with the doona or blankets, but from my experience I have to say there was never a time when anything like this occurred. The baby is right next to you, part of your subconscious brain is connected to them, and any sense that something is not as it should be will wake you up. Some people call this intuition. Research has shown that babies and mothers who co-sleep develop the same sleep rhythms.

However, it is definitely not safe to have a baby in a bed where two double beds are pushed together to make a large King size bed as there is a very big risk that the baby may slip down between the beds. Nor is it safe for the baby to be in the bed with parents who are under the influence of drugs or alcohol, as the risk of harming them is increased greatly through being in an altered state of awareness. Neither should a baby share a bed with a smoker. Other warnings about co-sleeping include avoiding a waterbed and making sure the baby does not get over-heated.

Another point to note about having a baby in the bed with you is that should the covers go over a baby's face their automatic response is to start wriggling their head and moving their arms around to get it off them. As Sheila Kitzinger writes in her book, *Breastfeeding Your Baby*:

There is no danger of suffocation for a healthy baby in a big bed – he will turn his head from side to side and move away if something blocks his nostrils and prevents him from breathing.

As a mother who has fed all of her babies night after night in the bed, I feel the greatest benefit for both mother and baby is that the baby does not get over-stimulated at night. A normal scenario for me would be this: before I go to bed I would sit in an armchair and feed off the left breast. Then I would carry the baby to bed and tuck us both up for the night, lying the baby on a towel in the middle of the bed. When the baby awakes for the next feed around midnight, all I have to do initially is find my little soft torch, turn it on, gain correct attachment and breastfeeding begins. The baby and I then fall back to sleep.

For the early morning feed around 3 a.m. I would pull the baby across the bed on the towel, to my left breast side. The reason I used a towel was so as not to arouse and excite the baby in any way. I would then breastfeed off the left breast, and when finished would slide the baby back into the middle of the bed once again. By always returning the baby to the middle of the bed I could then get back to sleep, as I could relax knowing my baby was not going to roll off.

One of the reasons I always had a baby on a towel was to prevent picking my baby up during the night. Picking a baby up, changing their nappy during the night and using a bright light to breastfeed will get a baby excited and really awake, which can make it very difficult to settle back down to sleep once the breastfeed is over. The less stimulation the better. I feel this teaches babies that the darkness and lack of stimulation means sleep time, which invariably suggests that there is a difference between night and day.

One mother told me that in order not to have to change a nappy in the night all you have to use is a good disposable nappy. Choose a brand that has the capacity to holds lots of urine and one that draws the urine through the layers away from the baby's skin, so they can last the whole night through.

Every co-sleeping family will work out what's best for them. Mothers can always experiment to find the right night-time routine for them. Some women roll their babies over at night to feed from the other breast. Other mothers shift their own body so that the 'top' breast is more accessible to the baby than the 'lower' breast (of course this indicates you have rather large breasts if you can feed from the top breast while you are lying on your side). It is even possible to feed twins in bed at night without disturbing them too much.

Initially, some mothers start off doing night-time feeds in a comfy armchair, even falling asleep with the baby until the next feed. The advantage of sitting up to feed initially is that it is easier to pay attention to good latching when you are learning to breastfeed. On the other hand, feeding lying down while the baby is drowsy can help the baby use its natural reflexes to latch on. Remember that if something doesn't work one week, it may work the next week, as babies are always changing. And you are always changing too, as you keep trying new things until you find what works best for you as the mother and baby pair.

Tips For Mothers With Newborns

- A great way to settle a baby down for a sleep in the daytime is to lay them onto a bunny rug/wrap that you have previously slept on. This is because it will have your smell on it and the baby will feel more settled as they can smell you nearby. Try not to get breast milk on the bunny rug/wrap though, as all they may want to do is feed.

- Buying a sling and having lessons in how to use it is essential. Once you have mastered the art of using a sling you will love it. Using a sling enables a baby to lay down horizontally for a breastfeed, which can be a lifesaver if you are out shopping and want to breastfeed discreetly. A sling is also very helpful if you or your partner want to take a walk or prepare your food and your little bub does not want to be put down. The sling is also great for dads to use, as they too can feel a closeness and bonding by having the baby close to their body.

- If your friends and family want to buy you a gift suggest that they buy you some nappy service. Nappy service will bring you any type of nappy and dispose of it for you the next week. For cloth nappies all you have to do is put them into the provided bin and they collect them and give you a new bin full of clean nappies. It saves a lot of time and energy washing nappies.

- During the final six weeks of pregnancy cook extra dinner food and freeze it. If your friends and family really want to assist you, have them bring meals around or have them cook for you. If you don't have family around save $20 a week while you are pregnant and find someone like a postpartum doula who will come into your home and prepare meals that can be eaten fresh or frozen. This can really take the pressure off a new mum.

- Have a cleaner come into your home and do the essentials on a daily basis. This can free you up to sleep when your baby sleeps, or to sit down and breastfeed, or to go out for a walk with the pram/sling or play with your baby.

- If things are really getting you down – get out of the house! Even if it seems too hard to get yourself and the baby out, make the effort. There is nothing that helps more than a change of scene, as well as the lovely comments you will get as people admire your cherub. If possible, get out and walk (baby in sling or pram), as the fresh air and exercise will change your mood immediately.

- For every difficult day you have, know there will be a great day where your little cherub will smile for the first time, or make a gurgling sound of joy, that will remind you of this precious gift you have brought into the world.

- If your baby is tired but is not settling, get into the bath with your baby. The warm water and skin-to-skin contact with your body can help to calm and soothe a restless baby. Just have your baby float gently on their back with you supporting them or have them lay on your chest with their body under the water. The bath is also an ideal place to breastfeed your baby in a relaxed, calm way.

- Really trust that you are doing the best possible job that you can, given your knowledge and skills. Unfortunately – or fortunately – a newborn baby does not come with a manual that states what we should be doing as a parent. Parenting/Mothering is very much an on-the-job learning experience that dictates we respond in any given moment the best way we know how. Try to stay calm and relax into your new role and honoured position of primary care provider for your beautiful baby, whom you created and brought into this world.

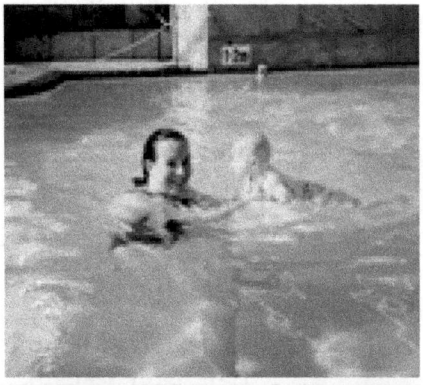

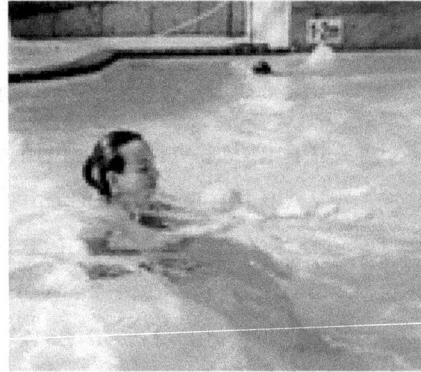

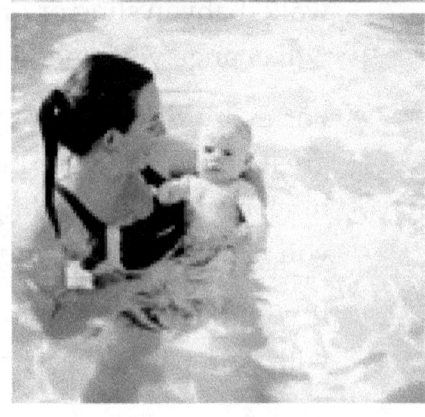

- Enrol your baby into swimming classes as soon as you can. Baby-swim is a wonderful way for babies to learn about water being a positive environment that should not be feared. The bonding between Mum, Dad and bubs is enhanced tenfold when in the pool as classes focus on lots of songs, games and water exposure, not forgetting the trust aspect. Early attendance at baby-swim classes assists in developing confidence in both the parents and baby, happy babies/ children who can rescue themselves and swim short distances should they need to within their first year of participation, hence it could make a big difference should they fall into water. It is a fact that is so important in Australia, particularly as so many people have backyard swimming pools.

25
Pregnancy Topics of Interest

The following pregnancy issues are ones that I felt compelled to address because they always arouse debate and feisty conversations during my antenatal classes. The information I have included here is based on my own beliefs and opinions, but of course I recommend you research these issues for yourself so that you can make your own informed opinion and decisions.

Listeria hysteria

The reason I have termed this disease *'listeria hysteria'* is because back in 1995 and 1997, when I was pregnant with my first and second babies, there was no mention or information about this infection at that time. By the time I was pregnant with my third baby in 1999, everywhere I turned and looked I was told 'you can't eat this, you can't eat that'! It was an hysterical approach to managing the risk of listeria, and all the foods that I had previously eaten to my heart's content during my first and second pregnancies were now forbidden.

Why the lack of information only nine years ago, and why all the panic now? Like myself, there were many women who just had no clue about foods containing listeria and we blissfully and contentedly ate our pate and Camembert, without an imaginary finger being pointed in disapproval.

So what is listeria? The listeria infection (listeriosis) is an illness caused by eating food contaminated with bacteria called listeria monocytogenes. Pregnant women are considered to be a high-risk group because when the listeria bacterial infection has entered the pregnant body through contaminated food, it can be transmitted to the foetus, causing miscarriage, stillbirth, premature birth or serious illness in newborn babies.

In some people listeria may present itself as a mild fever, headache, or just aches or pains like the flu. Others may show no signs at all, which makes it hard to detect. The incubation period is still very much unknown. If a pregnant woman suspects that she has been exposed to the infection it can be treated with antibiotics, which can kill the bacteria.

From health department pamphlets

Listeria grows best:

- on food stored for long periods of time (so clean out the fridge regularly).
- when food is prepared unhygienically in a kitchen (pre-wash cutting boards and food preparation areas thoroughly before making a meal).

The following food should be avoided if not freshly prepared and eaten within a twelve-hour period:

- home-made pate
- cooked chicken

- meat products, e.g. ham, and other manufactured meats
- soft cheeses, e.g. brie, Camembert, fetta and ricotta
- self-serve salads at a salad bar, or pre-packed salad packs, including coleslaw
- cold smoked and raw seafood, e.g. smoked salmon, oysters and sashimi
- soft-serve ice-cream and thick shakes

Ignorance is bliss, they say: I will vouch for that. However, was I right in being ignorant? Now, taking into account the current health warnings, I think that if pregnant women take it upon themselves not to get caught up in all the hype around listeria and eat home-cooked, healthy food that is washed and fresh, they will be on the right track. Using your initiative is the key to enjoying your favorite foods.

My tips

- Try to avoid food not prepared in your own kitchen, or food that has been handled by someone else.
- Heating food destroys the listeria bacteria, so if in doubt heat your food.
- Thoroughly wash all fresh fruit and vegetables as this can help remove the bacteria from the outside.

Group B Streptococcus

'Strep B' refers to the colonisation of the Streptococcus B bacteria in the vagina. If there is a high density of Strep B it greatly affects the natural vaginal flora, making it possible for the baby to be exposed to the Group B Streptococcus infection on its journey through the birth canal, which can cause a serious reaction in newborns.

Although women often have Strep B in their vagina at normal levels, it only poses a real problem around the time of labour and birth because this is the time that a baby can be exposed to this bacteria once the membranes have broken. The longer the membranes have been broken the greater the risk of exposure for a baby in utero.

In 'Infection in pregnancy', Elaine Wang and Fiona Smaill, state that:

> Group B strep has become the most frequent cause of overwhelming sepsis in neonates. The early and most serious form of infection is characterized by rapid onset of respiratory distress, sepsis and shock. The likelihood of disease (approximately 2 per 1000 live births) is directly related to the density of colonization and the immaturity of the infant. Infants with birth weights less than 2500 grams have a much higher overall infection rate than infants weighing 2500 grams or more. Pre labour rupture of the membranes and maternal fever are also associated with a higher incidence of infection.

Recent research shows that the protocols currently used for the prevention of a Strep B infection in a newborn are inconclusive. However, having said that, many women who have Strep B going into labour are offered antibiotics intramuscularly or intravenously every four hours, as this can reduce the transmission of Group B Strep.

Elaine Wang and Fiona Smaill, go on to state that:

> The available data show that a course of antibiotics given during pregnancy results in only a temporary eradication of group strep B carriage, with no detectable effects on infant colonization or sepsis with group B strep. Treatment during pregnancy, unless continued into labour, has only a transient effect on the vaginal flora and will not influence the rate of sepsis in the newborn.

An alternative to treating the mother who has Strep B is to treat the newborn at birth. Antibiotics can be given to neonates at the time of birth. A difficult decision will have to be made if you have a positive Strep B swab close to the time of birth. Will you have antibiotics during labour? Will you give the baby antibiotics in case it gets a serious Strep B infection? It is never an easy decision to give a newborn antibiotics, or even to have the baby tested for Strep B if the mother has a high-density ratio on or close to the birth-day.

The swab for detecting Strep B is performed by the woman herself, by rubbing an oversized cotton bud in her vagina and inside her anus at around thirty-six to thirty-eight weeks. (It does not paint a pretty picture does it – a woman trying to swab herself while heavily pregnant!) The swabs are then sent off for testing, which usually takes about two days. If the results come back positive an informed decision will need to be made as to whether or not you decide to have the antibiotics while in labour, and, if you decide you will, then which way you would like them administered. The choice is through injection (in the thigh or bottom) or through a bung (drip-intravenously). The downside to the latter method is that the medical care providers may want you to leave the bung in your hand, which can be very annoying. You do have a choice about this!

In order to test if a baby has been exposed to the antibiotics, the simplest and easy way is to swab inside a baby's ear canal. A swab can also be taken from the back of the throat or a gastric aspirate can be performed. This is where the contents of the baby's stomach are sucked out and sent off for testing. The downside to this is that it can leave a baby suffering from chronic reflux from the little sphincter valve the tube pushes past to get into the stomach becoming floppy and lax, which can result in stomach acids being secreted up the oesophagus. In the meantime, the results take a few days to come back, so antibiotics may have already been given regardless of whether the baby does or does not have Strep B.

I have attended many births where the labouring woman had Strep B and no antibiotics were offered to her or the newborn at that particular hospital, with no resulting health problems for mother and baby. I have attended births where the labouring woman has had four-hourly jabs in the bottom and the baby still had Strep B, with no signs or symptoms at all detrimental to the baby's health. I have attended births where women have had Strep B and the labouring woman has decided not to have antibiotics and the baby has been born with Strep B, but with no signs or symptoms detrimental to the baby's health. Then again, babies have died from this infection. How do you weigh up the risks of treatments and outcomes?

You can see how this topic raises intense discussion among women and medical professionals! This is very much one of the current hot issues, where an informed decision needs be made should the results be positive. If a woman's results come back negative or as a low-density ratio, she will not be faced with making a decision about Strep B.

An alternative point to note here is that my good friend and associate Faye has observed that when women have a lavender essential-oil bath prior to having their swab for Strep B, the results, more often than not, come back negative. Faye believes that lavender has the effect of balancing out the natural flora of the vagina, hence decreasing the percentage of Strep B to a low-risk level. I figure having a lavender bath is definitely worth consideration, so enjoy!

Glucose Tolerance Test For Gestational Diabetes

I feel compelled to include this information as often women undergo these tests not fully understanding what they are designed to indicate, or with no understanding of the possible outcomes of gestational diabetes.

The diagnosis of 'gestational diabetes' is based on an abnormal glucose test, which in Australia is detected through two tests. The first is the glucose challenge test. The woman is asked to drink a fifty-gram concentrate of glucose solution and has her blood taken one hour later. If all appears within the normal range she will not be asked to come back to do the glucose tolerance test.

The glucose tolerance test is where a woman is asked to fast for eight hours, then has her blood taken, drinks a seventy-five gram concentrate of glucose, then two hours later has another blood test. If it appears that her blood glucose is high, it is assumed that her body has not sufficiently metabolised the glucose properly, hence has gestational diabetes.

Is there a real problem with having gestational diabetes? Can it affect the baby and the birth? How does it affect the mother?

As Hunter and Kierse explain:

The 'adverse outcome' most frequently associated with gestational diabetes is 'fetal macrosomia' (a larger than average baby). The adverse outcomes of caesarean section, shoulder dystocia and trauma derive from this primary outcome. Up to 30 per cent of mothers with an abnormal glucose tolerance test have a baby with a birthweight of more than 4000 grams. However, clinical judgement based on assessment of pre-pregnant weight, weight gain and a pregnancy past 42 weeks, without any reference to glucose tolerance, is more predictive of fetal macrosomia than is the glucose tolerance test. Wide application of glucose tolerance testing to pregnant women would thus be of limited value in identifying women at increased risk of fetal macrosomia.

Hunter and Keirse also go on to state that:

... there is no convincing evidence that treatment of women with an abnormal glucose-tolerance test will reduce perinatal mortality or morbidity. Trials of dietary regulation for 'gestational diabetes' do not demonstrate a significant effect on any outcome, including macrosomia. Trials comparing the use of insulin plus diet with diet alone show a decrease in macrosomia, but no significant effect on other outcomes such as use of caesarean section, the incidence of shoulder dystocia, or perinatal mortality. There is also no evidence that such treatment reduces the incidence of neonatal jaundice or hypoglycemia.

So the likelihood of a baby dying from gestational diabetes is very small. The main outcome of gestational diabetes is that your baby will be larger (for example, the fundus may measure twenty-six centimetres when you are only twenty-two weeks pregnant). The worst-case scenario for women who have bigger babies is shoulder dystocia (they get wedged) when coming out. There could be a genuine need for a Caesarean if it is a huge baby (keeping in mind that Caesareans also have risks). I consider 'huge' to be over ten pounds. Diet can assist with keeping the baby's weight down and exercise should be a part of everyday life, even if just a walk. Gestational diabetes treatment does not affect neonatal jaundice or hypoglycemia.

Many times I have had women return to my antenatal classes after they have been told that they have gestational diabetes. One young, fit, healthy woman came to my class in tears. When I asked her what the trouble was she replied, 'I have gestational diabetes and the doctor told me that I have to go on a strict diet and stop being a pig and eating lots of food, because my baby is too big for my body.' This particular woman really took to heart her doctor's words and reduced her food intake to the extreme. She only ate when she really had to, if at all, terrified of having a big baby. As she went along over the next trimester of her pregnancy, her doctor kept planting the seed of her inability to be able to birth naturally due to the baby's likely size. He did not address the fact that her health was failing due to lack of sufficient nutrition. When the doctor had won outright and this baby was born via a Caesarean section, the baby weighed a little over five pounds, hardly a big baby by anyone's estimate!

Like all pregnancy and birthing issues, women do have a right of choice about whether or not to have a glucose test in the first place. And there are alternative tests, such as a simple skin-prick test on your finger.

In Summary

During pregnancy there are so many things that women need to be aware of and make choices about that it is almost overwhelming at times. For this reason, I suggest that you listen to your gut instinct on any such matters, as well as reading articles and books about the actual issues and details and, more importantly, the likely outcomes for you and your baby. Really tune into yourself and your body and see what it is saying. Self-intuition is a powerful thing if you take the time to listen.

26

Birth Stories

I have asked some of the women I know to share their birth stories in this book, to inspire other women. Some of the births presented here are ones that I attended as a doula, and others I did not. The major purpose of these birth stories is to demonstrate and share how wonderful birth can be, regardless of whether the birth takes place at home, in a birth centre, hospital, or in the car on the way to hospital!

I did ask some of the women to try to highlight how they prepared for a positive natural birth experience, so that other readers could acknowledge what they need to do. Each story is unique and personal to the couple involved, therefore for privacy reasons I have changed the names of a few couples. I felt each of the stories I chose to include had an underlying message, lesson or informative guide to assist others to start to understand the intricacies of labour and birth.

I have included a range of birth situations in order for readers to gain a true feel for the events that lead up to a natural birth outcome. I hope that these stories do assist your desire to give birth naturally. Enjoy!

A Wonderful Birthing Experience

As I sit here and write this birth story, I look over and see my seven-month-old looking back at me with his beautiful big eyes. It is sometimes hard to believe that he grew inside of me and came out of me through a natural vaginal birth. He was a little over ten pounds in weight, rather a big boy out of my rather thin, small-framed body. How the time after you have a baby flies, it really does. I remember women saying to me to really enjoy this short, precious time with your baby, because before you know it they will be toddlers, running about.

Back to the birth. During my pregnancy I travelled along knowing that I would possibly be having a C-section. I thought this because all my friends with babies had had one, so I expected I would also. The only information or understanding I had about birthing came through these main friends of mine. I did have one other friend who told me about a doula who had attended her birth and how this person also ran aqua classes at the pool. With total amazement I learned about the one and only natural birth experience out of all my friends. Somehow a natural birth really started to appeal to me. So when I met Gaby through her antenatal classes at the pool I began to consider the possibility of not having a C-section. I felt I was being challenged about my belief systems every time I attended the class at the pool, and the concept, and my belief in my own ability to birth naturally, started to become a reality.

With only six weeks to go before my estimated birth-day, I asked Gaby to attend the birth of our baby. Gaby had been the doula for my friend, who'd had a big healthy boy naturally with no tear. This intrigued me, and I was reassured that women just like myself can birth in a natural way.

As the last six weeks went by I tried really hard to block out all of the really negative birth stories and outside influences and listen to positive birthing stories only. It was not long before I realised I could birth naturally if I wanted to, as there was nothing really stopping me making that decision. Over the next few weeks I invested my time wisely and tried to prepare myself mentally by learning specific labour/birthing meditations, visualisation and relaxation with Gaby. I also worked at physically preparing myself by attending the deep-water aqua running classes, toning relaxation aqua classes, and pregnancy-specific fitball sessions, all of which helped me to stay toned, aerobically fit and more flexible.

On my due date I went into labour at about four in the morning. At 7 a.m. I rang Gaby to let her know so she could plan her day. She came over for her usual 'check-in' session just to see where I was at and connect with me on various levels to suss out what exactly was going on. Gaby had explained to me that she would not stay for long if it looked like there was nothing really going on. This way I would be free to really go into labour without her watching me and possibly causing what she calls 'performance anxiety'.

As it turned out, I had a false start, and by 9 a.m. my contractions had completely stopped. As Gaby described it, nature had been really kind and had given me a taste of what labour actually feels like and a little introduction to warm-up labour. As planned, Gaby went home and I just plodded around the house doing a few jobs, trying to sit down and rest when I could. I actually had a reflexology appointment booked at 11 a.m. that I was determined to attend, so maybe this is why my labour stopped?

After attending the reflexology session, which really stirred everything up, I went home and jumped into bed to have a cat nap. As I lay there in the bed the contractions became stronger. The time was now 2 p.m. and Gaby arrived to find me half-asleep, moaning in the bed, unsure whether or not to get up or stay put. I decided I needed to get up as the intensity was definitely getting stronger the longer I lay there.

One of my biggest worries was about my waters breaking on the couch, as I thought the smell and mess would ruin it completely. So it came as a complete shock when my waters totally broke on the couch at approximately 2.30 p.m. in the afternoon. I guess 'our thoughts really do create our reality'! At that moment I jumped up to run to the bathroom and left a trail of amniotic fluid all the way through the house. As I stood in the shower still more fluid came out of my body. I said to Gaby, 'Geez, how much of this stuff comes out?' I just could not believe how much there was. In fact I was sure that it was at least a bucketful. I left Gaby and my husband to the unenviable task of mopping up, while I stayed in the shower to labour away. Things were happening now and I knew this was the real thing.

After a major clean-up, including the couch, which we all laughed about, Steve assisted me back to the lounge room, where I sat on a fitball, then I moved to the bed on my hands and knees. I tried to get comfortable but felt restless so Gaby suggested a walk around the block. It was almost dark at this stage so it didn't bother me to be labouring away outside. I just needed some air. Before Gaby and I headed off I had some Rescue Remedy, which really helped to keep me calm.

At 10 p.m. we all decided it would be a great idea to head for the hospital as the contractions were really getting strong. The only problem was that one of the worst storms to hit Perth in ten years was occurring, as we got into the car to drive from Fremantle to Mount Lawley, a forty-minute drive. It was an interesting trip to say the least. I laboured away very peacefully, unaware that the water from the Swan River was being thrown over our car, as lightning flashed overhead and the thunder roared. Steve just turned up the Pachelbel's Canon louder to drown out the noise. And I was in labour heaven, oblivious to all of this – well, sort of, I was aware but not aware. Steve decided we would call our baby 'Thor', after the god of thunder!

Arriving at the hospital, I got into the shower to warm up and relax a little after our trip. This gave Gaby the chance to fill up the bath tub, which I was dying to get into. All was going well till the lights went out! A complete blackout of the hospital occurred while I was standing in the shower in a small bathroom with the door closed. Thankfully, the midwife was able to locate a torch to come and check on us to see if we were fine. I figured it was just as easy to stay put and not move, as I was happy where I was. It did take a good while before the lights actually came back on, after which we had to put up with alarms going off, bells ringing and all sorts of buzzers for the rest of the night. Finally, I stepped into the tub. It really was as great as I had heard it would be. Instantly I sank down and relaxed. Gaby talked me through a few meditations whereby I actually slept in between my contractions. I stayed in the tub for four hours (as I learned the next day), and yet it seemed like it was only half an hour to an hour tops. I was really surprised to learn that information. Birth hormones really do distort the way a woman in labour perceives the time.

After the four hours in the tub I started to feel a little urge to push, and wanted to go to the toilet, so I hopped out of the tub. I felt instantly very cold and shivery, so Gaby and Steve raced around to get me some clothes I could throw on, as well as socks to keep my feet warm. After a while I started to feel much warmer, and with the help of more Rescue Remedy I remained calm and focused.

Gaby had prepared the room by getting a mattress for the floor, with a big beanbag and lots of pillows, and it was here that I continued to labour away. After a period of time labouring and feeling like I wanted to push but couldn't, I opted for a vaginal examination to see what was going on. It was at this stage I found out I had an anterior lip, so I needed to stop pushing and breathe through, to try to assist it to push over, away from the baby. For the next twenty minutes I breathed and panted my way through lots of contractions. It was bloody hard work!

After another internal where the midwife actually flicked the lip away, I was able to start pushing my baby out of my body. It was now that I started to feel the full extent of hormonal activity as I again began to feel restless and wanted to move about in between the contractions – when I squatted holding on to the back of a chair. When each pushing urge was over I would then stand up and walk around the room. I was a woman on a mission, possessed by mother nature. Nothing was going to stand between me and my baby. I was getting pissed off now and demanding to know how much longer, as little by little my baby moulded his head down and through my body. It was hard work but rewarding work, as I could start to feel the movement downwards towards mother earth.

The midwife I had at this point had been with me all night and had stayed over her shift to assist me the best way she knew how. She was really brilliant as she honoured me in every way, by accepting Gaby's presence at the birth and reassuring Steve. We were a team effort, all working towards the same goal and purpose. The only time I felt pressure to be doing something the 'right way' or more quickly was when my ob (obstetrician) came into the room demanding to know if the baby really was moving down. As if we had conspired to make up the story! He demanded the midwife be accountable and truthful, and he just looked at Gaby as if to say, 'And who the hell are you?' It was an interesting turnaround in every conceivable way from the wonderful supportive night that I had just had.

The pressure was on me now to get up on the bed, as my ob was not happy with the length of time I had been pushing. Thankfully, when I hopped onto the bed my baby's head was sitting just under my perineum, and so my ob assisted my baby out, trying to prevent a tear to my perineum. Although I was on my back with my legs up I did find this position helped to really push my baby out. Having my feet firmly on someone, pushing, seemed to give me an extra bit of energy and strength.

After sixteen hours of labour I brought into the world the most beautiful big baby boy, who was over ten pounds, with just a little tear and no painkillers at all. All I could think about after the birth was, I did it, I really did it, and I couldn't wait to tell my friends and family about my wonderful experience. I really felt alive and like I could do anything and handle any situation from that day forward. Thanks to the help of Gaby I achieved the type of birth I set out for, in every way possible. I say never underestimate what the presence of another woman with you at your birth can do.

I truly believe that having Gaby attend our birth allowed me to relax, enjoy and therefore focus on breathing through the contractions and relaxing. As a result of doing this I didn't once feel as though I needed any form of pain relief. Steve was just able to focus on me and the birth and not worry about other issues like what to do or when to say something.

Birth Story For Baby Luci Alyce

Back in early March, Gary and I decided it was time to stop being selfish and start a family. Luckily for us it wasn't so difficult and before we knew it I was pregnant. I felt I knew from day one that all was 'go' – my body just told me all was okay and the baby-making process was underway.

My profession is an aerobics instructor/personal trainer, so monitoring my heart rate was most important to me. I cut down on my cardio classes, especially the high-impact ones, and concentrated on the toning.

I went through my pregnancy very easily, but could not believe how much energy it used up. From being a person who was hyper and always on the go, I found it hard to slow down.

Now, looking back, Thursday was a big day. It started at 5 a.m. supervising in the gym, followed by a two-hour walk through Kings Park, including the Kokoda trail, back to the gym for lunchtime supervision followed by a circuit class in which the 'hula hoops' came out. Watching the participants wiggle those hips and try and keep the hoop up was so much fun – the laughing and banter was alive! Mid-afternoon I was on my way home – rather tired but with more to do that day. Waxing was next priority, followed by the weekly shop and home to unload. Deciding that we were just too tired to cook, Gary and I took off for an early dinner at the local Indian. After a tasty meal it was home to bed, it had been a long day and sleep was needed.

Well, the sleeping soon ceased at about 10.30 p.m. All of a sudden I felt like I had lost control of my bladder, so I bolted out of bed not realising what was going on (this was all happening three weeks early!). Did the toilet thing and then back to bed, but no sooner had I got comfortable and it happened again. You know how 'everyone' tells you that in first pregnancies the baby never comes early – well don't listen. I realised then what was going on, that labour was starting, but went to the toilet again just to be sure. Now the other thing that 'everyone' tells you is that first pregnancies are prone to a long labour – again, not always true. I went back to bed and lay there looking at the clock trying to time my contractions, which were coming in four- to five-minute intervals. Within the hour they were only minutes apart, so I thought it was time to wake Gary.

It was amazing how quickly he moved. After weeks of me being hassled over packing my bag for the big day, guess who didn't have his packed? So the panic was on!

By midnight the contractions were coming hard and fast and with a quick call to the Family Birthing Centre (FBC) we needed to be on our way. Well that was easier said than done – trying to run between contractions when I could feel the baby bearing down was a challenge in itself. It took twenty minutes before I was kneeling in the front seat of our VW Polo (facing the back) and Gary zoomed off down the street. Six red lights and a section of roadworks later, our gorgeous little girl, Luci Alyce, was born in the car outside Karrakatta Cemetery. Of all the places to be born, it was outside the cemetery!

Yep, she was in a hurry, and in that much of a hurry she came out bum first. It was scary – birthing her myself was one thing, but when I realised I had her bum in my hand, that was something else. Then the feet came out. I started to worry about where that cord was going to be. I yelled at Gary to stop the car, which he did, and he came around to the passenger side. When he got there, I told him to hold 'this' – he did not realise just what 'this' was! It was our baby's legs and bottom. I tried to reposition myself and feel where the cord was going, as my biggest worry was it was going to be around the baby's neck. Then the penny dropped for Gary, who assessed the urgency of the situation and said that we needed to get to the FBC. Luckily, I finally felt the cord was free of Luci's neck and when Gary took off, in a bit of a panic, out she popped!

Arriving at the FBC I was now seated properly on the front seat with our gorgeous little girl in my lap still attached. As the door opened at the birth centre, Gary fell into the midwife's arms with all that had just happened, as it started to sink in. The mid wife who greeted my husband at the door was Wendy, who came to the car to assist me into the birth centre. I said to her that Luci had come out bum first – 'no,' she said, 'that can't be right', but then her eyes popped out of her head as she saw the big pressure bruise on Luci's bottom. It was time to move from the car to inside where I stumbled about awkwardly, Luci still connected to me via the umbilical cord. I attempted to get onto the bed, where I sat in a state of contemplation and shock from the speed in which I had just birthed. The midwives allowed me (us) to stay like that for about twenty minutes, letting us all get over the shock of our experience.

Luci was then freed and put under a heat lamp while I was brought a cup of tea and waited for the placenta to make its debut. Another twenty minutes passed and all was over – now it was time to relax and take it all in.

After all the reading I had done in the nine months, everything that I had been told seemed so irrelevant now. I know that I didn't have the 'norm' kind of birth but I did feel that perhaps too much emphasis is put on the educational part of labour and not enough emphasis is placed on the aftercare. Being a first-time mum I had not had exposure to many babies before and a little terror set in, knowing that I was now a parent. All of a sudden the responsibility of this tiny, helpless human is yours – don't get me wrong, it is wonderful, but scary at the same time.

I could not have asked for better support from the FBC – the midwives and the environment get you ready for normal life ahead. It was off home just before 6p.m. and this time there was three of us. The experience was wonderful and I am ready to do it all again, but maybe not in the car!

The Beautiful Birth of Gala

When friends without children ask me if labour hurts I don't really know what to say. Childbirth is different for every woman. I have a friend who gave birth in an hour and a half and once her child was in her arms she said, 'I don't know what all the fuss is about!' I believe I could probably enlighten her. With two average-length births (approximately twelve hours) under my belt I must confess the pains of labour are excruciating. However, I must also declare that with proper education, support and physical and mental preparation, it is a pain that is bearable.

We women are made of stronger stuff than fluff. My first birth experience was in a hospital. I had decided I wanted a natural childbirth without an epidural. During pregnancy, though I kept myself physically fit, I did not participate in any pregnancy related classes. In fact I avoided them. But I chose to be in the hospital as I wasn't confident with the other options.

Having started contractions at 7p.m. and arriving at the hospital at 11p.m., by 5a.m., after numerous offers from the midwife, I opted for the epidural. The hospital staff all did their utmost to ensure the safe birth of my beautiful ten pound four ounce little boy, and at 7.30a.m. he came into the world. (The obstetrician who delivered him stayed back to complete the delivery after a twenty-four-hour shift.)

The baby was perfect and I was ready for visitors by 9 a.m. but I had a niggling feeling, which would only increase with time, that I had failed. I gave birth on my back, with my legs in stirrups, nurses pushing on my belly, in a room that looked like a dental surgery; not a homely environment. I had succumbed to the epidural and didn't have the presence of mind to ward off a huge episiotomy (leading to third-degree tearing). Though this may sound like kindergarten compared with what some women undergo, it was not how I'd imagined giving birth. In fact I didn't feel as though I'd done anything, as I felt my baby had been delivered by the swarm of medical professionals who'd surrounded me and then buzzed off never to be seen again once the babe arrived. I felt powerless.

On discovering I was pregnant for the second time I immediately started looking for antenatal fitness classes. I was only six weeks pregnant when I started Gaby's classes, but already, like those really annoying students at school who always made the class stay back after the bell had gone, I had a million questions. Second time round, I was determined to go through a labour without an epidural, and empowered.

We (my husband and I) opted on one of Western Australia's excellent birthing centres. I was doing antenatal aqua, antenatal yoga, antenatal meditation and active birthing classes, and had they offered antenatal nose-picking I'm sure I would've thrown myself into that as well. I decided I might need extra help, and into the third month Gaby agreed to be my doula. I already knew I had made the right choice but my husband and mother (the rest of the support team) needed convincing. My mother, a registered nurse who had studied midwifery, was sceptical about the role of the doula. She saw it as taking over the midwife's role and needed a little convincing of Gaby's function.

The four of us had three meetings before the birth and Gaby and I spoke together numerous times during and after the aquatic classes at the pool. We spoke about whatever was concerning me at the time: fear of tearing, fear of having a girl, standing up to doctors, how to have the Strep B administered, when to call her, etc.

At week thirty-nine I felt very fit and everything was ready to go. The baby's head had been down for three months, but my appointment with the midwife revealed that it had turned and was in a transverse position. The midwife started using the 'C' word and I almost broke down into tears on the spot (not that it's unusual for a heavily pregnant woman). I spoke with Gaby before my ultrasound and she assured me the baby would probably be back in the head-down position by the next day. Sure enough, at the ultrasound the bub was back head-down. It was a valuable episode as it revealed my true fears and with the help of Gaby allowed me to let go of them.

Week forty-one, the morning of 10 April, I started contractions and I knew it was go. I called Gaby at 7 a.m. to let her know things had started but there was no hurry. Maybe it's the same with all women but I thought I was closer than I was. When Gaby arrived around nine and showed no urgency I knew I could relax. I went outside, had contractions, called my sisters, had contractions, made muffins, had contractions, my husband polished everyone's shoes, including Gaby's, and I had contractions. With every contraction Gaby or my husband came and gave me a back rub and kept my hot-pack hot.

By 11.30a.m. all I could think of was the big bath at the birthing centre so I decided to move there. I was calling the shots. What a difference to my previous birth where I had been a slave to hospital protocol. We got to the birthing centre, only to find I had to come back into the real world for a time, to answer questions from the midwife. Then I argued with the doctor on how to administer my antibiotics for the Strep B. Though I give the doctor credit for being persistent, I won. I admit that doctors work incredibly hard, but they know about medicine and I know about me. Their knowledge must be balanced along with the understanding that a pregnant woman is not necessarily sick or stupid.

My husband, mother and son arrived just as the bath was filled. My husband and I got into the bath and time became liquid. We had music, oil and after a few suggestions from Gaby she left us to ourselves. The contractions hurt but in between I felt divine, nurtured – truly, I felt like a goddess. I'd never imagined that birthing could be this way. When my husband left, Gaby or my mum came in. They performed perfectly as a team to help me give birth in the way I chose.

When the midwife changed over at 4p.m., the time came for an internal. I thought I was nine or ten centimetres dilated, and when I found out it was five centimetres some quick words from Gaby stopped me from being self-piteous and helped me get on with it. At about this stage with my previous child I had taken the epidural. The two hours that remained seemed an eternity.

I was due a booster jab of antibiotics for the Strep B but at 5 p.m. I decided to pretend to start pushing so they wouldn't give it to me as I didn't really feel it was necessary to have another hit of antibiotics. Well, I did have a tiny urge to push, but at the same time I was scared to do so. This was the part where I had given my power over to the medical profession beforehand, and now I was the main player. I knew I had good support behind me to do what was needed: a great midwife, my husband, Gaby the super doula, my mum, and even my one-year-old.

The pain was like nothing I have experienced. I tore (but the tear was small) and I felt nothing but a burst of heat. And the sensation of suddenly feeling that head clunk into the pelvis was bizarre and marvellous. I am so grateful I was able to experience it. The intangible pains of contractions changed in an instant to an awareness that my baby was so close to revealing itself. And when she arrived I was exuberant, exhausted and still able to get up and walk to our room. My recovery was much faster. I had no grogginess. I had complete consciousness of my muscles and parts.

I felt empowered and strong.

My mother later commented that she saw the reason and place in having a doula – that it seemed to make everything more fluid. My husband said the support we found in her was the missing link. And as a side comment, my recovery from a drug-free birth was much quicker and I felt like I bounced back into life at home very easily.

Is that a leopard in your pants!

(Written by Gaby Targett, doula for Bronwyn and Michael. Edited/ Additional notes by Bronwyn Bell.)

Bronwyn contacted me to discuss her concern about not having the right support around her for the type of birth experience she would like. This, from a doula's perspective, is often the case, and where other medical professionals fear to go for litigation reasons. Hence, I came to be Bronwyn's birth-support person, along with her husband Michael, at King Edward Hospital in Perth. The following story is about sheer determination, strength and courage on Bronwyn's part to experience a very positive and powerful labour and birth experience from an Insulin Dependent Diabetes/VBAC (Vaginal Birth After Caesarean) perspective.

Going into this experience with Bronwyn, we had many discussions and birth ideas/plans being created. Right from the outset, I knew that Bronwyn had the strength of character to make her dream come true of having a vaginal birth, and she also had the will to succeed. How she made this possible was by going straight to the head honcho of the hospital, who was Dr Michael Humphrey (Director of Obstetric & Gynecological Clinical Care Units). It was here that she clearly stated what she wanted and how she wanted the staff to assist and support her and not hinder her in any way when she went into labour. Bronwyn asked for this appointment to clear up any misunderstanding from her perspective, as prior to this she had met with the general medical staff to present her ideal birth plan, and was told point-blank that having a VBAC as a person living with diabetes was out of the question, and furthermore, 'You have to be kidding, don't you?' A response that was not appreciated at all.

So this is where the need came from to research, investigate and educate ourselves about other women who had been in the same predicament, and how they went about making their choices based on their findings. Why shouldn't a woman be allowed to go into labour as a VBAC diabetic if she so chooses?

First and foremost, a woman having VBAC has to go into labour naturally, as she will not be induced due to the risk of rupture of the uterine wall. Secondly, research shows that living with diabetes significantly increases the risk of the baby dying in utero if the mother chooses to go past the forty-week duration of gestation. That leaves a woman in this position with few options, and Bronwyn decided she had one chance and that she was going to go into labour naturally prior to the forty-week mark. This is easier said than done!

Armed with the right people behind her and the most outstanding understanding, education and information about the hospital's policy and procedures (of just what was and was not going to be allowed), Bronwyn urged her body to go into labour naturally. How, you might ask? Well, Bron had acupressure, acupuncture, homeopathic remedies, reflexology, raspberry-leaf tea, sex and more sex, hot, hot curry, followed by the last-ditch attempt at week thirty-nine and six days: castor oil with an orange-juice chaser. Yuck, you might say, but 'A woman's got to do what a woman's gotta do!' On the day of the scheduled C-section, Bronwyn went into labour naturally.

From the moment I was with Bronwyn labouring I could see the determination in her eyes. This was a woman who really trusted her body and was determined to give labour a go. So for this reason Bronwyn decided to stay at home for the first part of her labour, moving about from the shower to the lounge-room floor, to the chair and back to the shower. All while she wore her lovely leopard-print pads in her undies! – something I had never seen before, which kept us laughing all night and into the next day. It was a funny sight to see this leopard-skin fabric positioned so perfectly, to say the least. Maybe these pads were a metaphor for who she is and what she represented. The cat of all cats, strong, proud and fearless in her quest for success!

In the early hours of the morning we all decided that we would head off to King Edward for the next leg of the journey. Here we were welcomed with a mix of anticipation and relief in a positive way. All the staff entering the room totally honoured Bronwyn, Michael and myself for what we were doing. This was, of course, to assist Bronwyn in any way we could. I make no mistake in saying that we were clearly doing what it seemed no one else had done before. There was a lot of 'hoo haa' initially.

However, once the staff settled in and read the head honcho's letter in Bron's file, which briefed the staff to leave us to our own devices as much as possible, everyone seemed to calm down and the staff took on a wonderfully supportive role.

Bronwyn spent the entire day moving from the bath, to the shower, to the birth ball, back to the shower, back to the room and back to the shower. Hour after hour she laboured away with the strongest desire and focus I have ever seen. Hour after hour Michael and I took Bronwyn's blood glucose levels, fed her food and drink and assisted with insulin when she needed it. Not once was she pushed or asked to do something she didn't want to do – to the credit of the staff and the hospital, they supported Bronwyn in every way possible.

After twenty-two hours of established labour Bronwyn asked to go on an insulin drip due to ketones building up within her body. At this stage it was also necessary to monitor the baby's heartbeat and a battery-operated heartbeat monitor was strapped to Bron's body so she could still move about. Yes, battery-operated foetal monitors do exist and prevent women needing to get onto the bed. Bronwyn had thoroughly researched this option and requested this form of monitoring if and when necessary. The staff (no doubt relieved) happily assisted in making this possible.

If anyone deserved to have a natural birth vaginally it was Bronwyn, but unfortunately dilation of the cervix was slow and the baby's head was still high and Bronwyn was running out of steam. After much deliberation with myself, Michael and the obstetrician, Bronwyn decided that she had done everything possible to have a natural vaginal birth. With a few tears shed by everyone, Bron decided she had given the labour a good go and as much as she wished otherwise, opted to have a C-section after a night and day of labour.

Bronwyn had a big baby boy weighing at 4940 grams at 7.39 p.m. on the evening of Saturday 2 August 2003. I believe this is such a wonderful story because Bronwyn demonstrated how women can beat the odds and plan to have a powerful birth experience, an experience that is not considered the norm. With lots of preparation, a strong will and a belief in what you really want, you can achieve and create anything.

What was most important about Bronwyn's birth was that this time around she had choices and the opportunity to experience firsthand what labour actually feels like, and to be honoured during this experience and treated normally with regard to her diabetes. Although the outcome was not what Bronwyn and Michael wanted, it was still a positive experience, as the journey was the focus, and it was one that Bronwyn is grateful for.

Bronwyn's Notes

Jack's birth was truly a powerful fulfillment and wish come true. All I wanted was to have a choice at all times, and I did achieve that, though often I had to heavily back each choice with educated response based on my research, but it was worth it.

I spent my last hours of my first pregnancy crying and feeling so totally disempowered and disappointed with no choice or say in what I wanted. The second time I spent those last hours labouring and it was a real joy for me to do so. I made the choice to have no drugs up until the epidural for the C-section, and for this I am truly grateful. The hormonal surges I felt in my labour state were a pleasure to experience and I am positive my baby loved the exposure to these hormones as well.

Jack was born with no need for the special-care nursery as his blood glucose readings were in the normal range (both almost unheard of for babies of diabetic mums). I believe because of my determination to go to forty weeks (or earlier if bub had decided so) my baby had the best possible postpartum chances. I also expressed milk daily a week prior to the forty-week date in case there was a necessity to compfeed (a top-up feed). I am very grateful to Gaby for her very attentive support, time and skills, which really helped Michael and I believe in this dream of experiencing labour and birth. Our journey was very powerful and a wonderful story to recount for other women and couples who may be facing a VBAC situation, with or without diabetes.

A Birth Story of A Different Kind

(Written by Gaby Targett, who was a doula for this couple.)

This couple, Sam and Ken, came to ask for support during the birth of their second child because of their traumatic first experience during childbirth. The first birth experience was truly the 'cascade of intervention' at its best. It was the usual story of induction, followed by the need to have an epidural as the contractions were just too painful, and then a long time on the bed on her back unable to move. When finally fully dilated, the baby was stuck, the mother was unable to feel the contractions or the need to push, so the baby was assisted out with forceps. In the process of having a forceps delivery, the coccyx bone was broken and a third-degree tear resulted after an initial episiotomy! Four toes (the mother's) were also broken due to the force with which this woman was asked to bear down and push doing a valsalva manoeuvre, pushing against the midwife's body.

As you can see, the first birth experience was not a pretty picture, and for obvious reasons there was a lot of fear and stress going through the second pregnancy, thinking that at the end of the road the same story could repeat itself.

When I came into the picture it was with welcome arms, and after a period of time I felt a wonderful rapport with this couple, who totally trusted and accepted what I had to say about the previous experience. Because of this trust, I was able to assist this couple to debrief and clear away the old baggage, cleaning the slate ready for the next birth experience.

After many visits to the house and lots of contact during the aqua-specific pregnancy classes, the arrival day was near. The three of us prepared the final touches to the birth plan. At the top, in really big writing, was written, 'A doula and my husband will be supporting me, to help me focus and stay really strong, as I give birth to my baby naturally with no assistance from anyone else.' This was Sam's objective.

At last the telephone call came from Sam's husband, Ken, at 11 p.m. in the night.

'Hi Gaby, it's Ken. Sam has gone into labour. I am trying to get her in the car but I am finding it really hard as she is making lots of noise and she doesn't want to move. I'll be at your house in ten minutes when I have got her in the car.'

Well, thirty minutes passed by in a flash and still no car. I decided to phone just to see if Ken needed me to help out in some way, after all they only lived across our park. When I rang Ken said, 'I now have Sam in the car as well as our son, I'm grabbing the bag now and I'll be over in one minute.' True to his word, Ken pulled up to a halt a minute later with a screech of the brakes.

I opened the door to find Sam on the back seat, half laying down, half seated with one leg in the air on the headrest and one on the floor. Sam was panting and groaning like an animal, all while her son sat happily in his car seat with big wide eyes observing in a bemused way. The first thing I suggested was for Sam to turn around and kneel on the back seat looking out the back window. At least then she could open up her knees and take the pressure off her coccyx bone and pelvis while I massaged her back. Relieved to be in a better position, we took off for the twenty-minute drive to the birthing centre.

At the halfway mark of our journey Sam started to mention the fact that she felt the urge to push a poo out and the urge was getting stronger and stronger with every contraction. Being the 'I'll do anything to support you' type of doula, I happily suggested, 'Oh, just go ahead, if you have the urge to push a poo just do it, I will catch it, no problems.' Well with that I lifted up Sam's dress to catch the imminent poo in my hands! Out it came before I could reach for a towel or open the window to throw it out. So now I was in a real predicament – not only did I know that what follows poo is a baby, but my hands were full of poo! Carefully I tried to rotate the window winder, to open the window enough to throw the poo out. After about two minutes of trying and thumb-cramping I was successful.

All the while Ken just cracked jokes and said 'It is OK, honey, we will just tell the car-hire people we didn't smoke in the car but we accidentally got poo on the seats during the birth of our baby!' With that, I completely lost the plot laughing, not to mention Sam, who was trying to say that she could not laugh because it hurt when she laughed. It was a very serendipitous moment and one which totally shifted the energy from fear and anxiety to a calm and 'we're OK' attitude. The only difficult part of this scenario was massaging Sam with the backs of my hands as she needed pressure on her back to cope with the intensity of her pain.

Finally we arrived at the birth centre, Sam just about ready to pop the baby out, Ken feeling relieved we had arrived, their son Santi wondering what all the fuss was about, and me with residue poo all over my hands.

The midwife took one look at me and said, 'You had better come this way with me and wash those hands.' It was a relief to be finally able to use my hands, and with that I moved into the birthing suite where Sam, Ken and Santi had been taken.

I suggested that Sam get onto a mattress on the floor to birth her baby. With that she not only went onto the floor, she lay on her side with her head completely under the bed, with her arm up and between the mattress and the base. It was here that she stayed for the remainder of her birth, which lasted all of about twenty minutes. During this time I could hear muffled sounds coming from her mouth, along with, 'Gaby, help me control what I do, don't let me tear, please.'

At this point I looked up to see both father and son sitting on the bed, observing quietly, in awe of Sam's strength and ability, as two midwives and myself assisted Sam to birth her baby. As Sam pushed her baby down onto her perineum her membranes exploded completely, flooding the floor around us, not to mention my pants from hip to foot! It was then that I stood up to hold Sam's leg up in the air, keeping her toes free from injury. With the help of the midwives we coached Sam's baby out through the perineum. Little by little she gently pushed and guided her baby without a tear. At last, Sam's nine and a half pound baby boy slipped gently and calmly from her body onto the floor.

Slowly, slowly, Sam moved her body out from under the bed to meet and greet her son face to face, skin to skin. Ken, Santi and the wonderful midwives and I were all laughing and crying and awash with emotion. The labour was fantastic, straightforward and wonderfully funny at times, leading to a positive birth experience. I was so privileged to have been a part of creating such a different experience from the first one, and honoured that they were open to changing their thoughts and feelings about birthing. Sam said afterwards, 'I was really ready to listen and open to preparing myself this time around, I really wanted a totally different experience and I got it.'

Everything that Sam had written on her birth plan (apart from the poo in my hands!) happened, and she was so thankful that she had been mentally prepared to turn her thoughts around to a more positive mindset. As for Santi, he just sat in amazement and awe of mum with her head under the bed giving birth!

What a doula did for us at our birth!

With my first and second births, I felt that I really didn't have the right support around me during my labour, apart from my husband, although he was not overly excited about another birth, as he didn't really want to see me go through the birth experience again. I had a friend and a non-communicative midwife present previously, both of whom offered me little to no support at all.

As a result of feeling that I had had no support or direction during both my first and second labours, I dreaded having to go through labour again. All I could remember and focus on were when the contractions started building up, the pain became unbearable, and I became very frustrated with everyone. As a result I ended up having a very negative experience that left me with bad injuries and a long recovery, in which I really felt traumatised.

When I fell pregnant with my third child I realised that I needed a professional support person, someone who could offer me emotional and continuous, connected support. A doula was the answer for me, and with little trouble I found Gaby, whom I had met during my previous pregnancies when I attended her antenatal classes at the swimming pool.

To me, a doula is a spiritual guide who looks after your spiritual, emotional and physical state during the lead-up to your birth, and most importantly during your labour and birthing of your baby. I feel that the birth of a baby is a very spiritual event, in which you are at your most vulnerable and yet connected in a way to your higher self, with the most amazing energy and inner knowing of the true forces of nature happening all at once. A doula, I felt, can nurture and protect your interests during this special time and make sure that the people around you support the type of birth you really want to have.

On the eve of my forty-week-plus-ten-days mark on the calendar, I had had enough. I was heavy, tired and fed-up. I rang Gaby to let her know that I had decided to go for an induction the very next day at 8a.m. Gaby, knowing herself the full extent of being over the, 'dare I say', EDD, knew exactly where I was coming from. She was very supportive, but suggested I have a bonk anyway just to see if I could get things going naturally. 'You have nothing to lose by trying!' With that exchange of words over the phone I poured a glass of champagne for my husband and I, and disappeared with him into our bedroom to give it a go.

Within half an hour of doing the 'wild thing' I was in labour. Completely in labour, to the point where I needed to phone Gaby back to let her know, but I found myself struggling to get to the phone. I went from nothing to contractions three minutes apart. I decided to head over to the hospital and meet Gaby there, as things were really happening.

After ten minutes of getting settled in our room, Gaby arrived, much to the relief of my partner, who at this stage was having recurring thoughts of our last experience at this same hospital. He was looking rather white around the gills.

Gaby suggested I get into the shower as she could sense I was working really hard on the contractions. For the next hour I worked in the shower, both standing and then sitting on the fitball, as the water pounded my back. Gaby massaged my back; this combined with the water sensation felt fantastic. I also opted for some gas that they had on a portable trolley that could be brought into the bathroom, which I was especially pleased about. After an hour I headed back to the birthing room, where I found myself wanting to get onto the floor on a mattress and lean over a beanbag with lots of pillows on top. It felt so calm and relaxing in this room as the light was soft and it was very quiet, except for the noises I was making. I stayed here to labour through to my transition stage, where I felt contraction upon contraction and again requested the gas for some relief. I also remembered throwing my head from side to side and asking,

'When is this baby coming!'

After a period of time my contractions seemed to disappear, giving me a complete break from the previous intensity I had felt. I almost felt like I had stopped labour and asked Gaby and the midwife, 'Why have they stopped?' Both Gaby and the midwife reassured me that it was OK for the body to take a break so it could get into gear for the pushing part. With that I felt a huge rush of hormones and heat as the need-to-push sensation came over my body like a wave. I knew that at last I was there, I had done what my body needed to do, which was to open up, and now all I had to do was push. The pushing part is hard. It takes real focus and determination. Thank goodness for the great hormones to help. The adrenalin helps to get really primal and go within. It also aided me in making lots of noise, which is something I feel assists in getting a baby out of your body.

I suddenly remembered to start listening to the midwife and Gaby, who by this stage were suggesting that I back off a little and not push so hard. I did feel like a woman possessed, on a mission, but I decided to stay focused and do as they suggested. My female obstetrician arrived at last to find me in the throes of giving birth, and just stood back to allow Gaby and the midwife to continue doing what they were doing. Slowly, little by little, I pushed my baby into the world. All the while my husband was up my head end giving me continuous support while Gaby and the midwife attended my vaginal and peri needs.

My aim was to keep my perineum intact as much as possible, even though I knew I was having a big third baby. I was over-joyed and relieved when my biggest baby, a boy weighing ten pounds four ounces, came sliding into the world and was caught by Gaby.

So, my third baby came out in three hours of labour, and I am writing this story to tell you there is such a thing as a *'beautiful birth'*, even with having a big baby, as I am living proof of that. I am not a big woman at all, in fact I am very small and petite, and yet I birthed a whopper baby. It truly is amazing what women can do when they are given the right mental preparation and emotional support during labour, and, above all else, the belief that they can birth their baby.

Birth Story By Alison

I consider my first and second birth experiences to be totally different. Of course, as with everything in life, we benefit from the experience of birth. However, I believe that had I been better prepared the first time, I could have had two positive birth experiences instead of one.

During my first pregnancy, I thought that being prepared and having a birth plan meant knowing how to breathe and what pain relief you wanted to have, if at all. Thus, I went into labour thinking I had an open mind about what was going to happen. So, when the midwife asked me, 'What is your birth plan?' I replied, 'I don't know what is going to happen, so I will decide as it happens.' I remember thinking how liberal I was going into labour without the assurance that I was going to have an epidural. I wanted a natural labour, but I also didn't know how painful it was going to be, so I thought I would leave my decision till later.

As I eventually found out during my second pregnancy, despite my confidence at the time of the first birth and despite all the reading I had done, I couldn't have been less prepared for what was to come first time around. Consequently, as the labour progressed and the pain gradually became worse, although I was handling it I know now that I was very afraid of the unknown and this fear slowed me down and shut my pelvis up tight. Despite this, I laboured through it and did not have any pain relief. I also had a terrible time pushing my baby out, and needed a vacuum extraction in the end. My memory of the labour was not positive afterwards (except for the reward being handed to me, which is indescribable). I therefore spent the next two years pitying pregnant women and was convinced that if I did it again, I would definitely have an epidural.

When I fell pregnant again, fate brought me to Gaby's classes when I was only fifteen weeks pregnant. I was drawn to the classes, looking forward to them and thirstily absorbing all the information and stories of other birth experiences. This journey not only prepared me for my second birth, but also helped me to see where I had gone wrong the first time. I was able to identify the fear that I had been carrying around with me and meet it head on, and therefore I was in a better place when the time came for the birth of my second child. I believe that even though I thought I was very prepared the first time round, it wasn't the right kind of preparation. The main things that I learned in the weeks leading up to the second birth were:

- that I was in full control of my own birth.
- that fear would make the pain far worse, and even halt the progress of labour.
- to ignore the negative stories and thoughts that other people love to dump on pregnant women all the time; just focus on the positive input (the end result could not be more positive!).
- be prepared with a birth plan when you walk into the hospital and share this birth plan with your obstetrician, midwives and support person/s before the birth.

Armed with this information, I had a great first stage of labour. I had known all day that I was going to have the baby soon, after having a significant bloody show in the morning and the beginnings of mild, irregular contractions (much like period pains). By the evening I was still able to cook dinner (with a few sit-downs) but I was beginning to distance myself from the insignificant chit-chat from the people around me and day-to-day routines, almost like being in a dream. I remember my mouth opening and closing to have a conversation with a visitor at our house, but I don't remember what I said. Eventually I knew I had to get away and so I went into the bedroom with my mum (who happens to be an aromatherapist) and she did shiatsu on me and massaged my abdomen and back. At this point I began to really relax and was now on a different planet altogether.

This experience was so different from the nervous excitement that I had felt the first time. This state of relaxed labouring continued into the night after everyone went to bed. I watched one of my favourite girlie movies, which I know practically by heart, and this helped to pass the time, while I continued to breathe through my contractions. Eventually I began to time them, my biggest concern being when to arouse my husband to go to hospital. At 3a.m. I started to feel pain in my back when having a contraction and in between contractions, and had to go on all fours. After a while I decided I needed to get into the shower. At this point my husband suggested that we go to hospital because they had a nice big bath, which we were keen to try.

Between making the decision and getting in the car, my contractions became closer together and more intense, so I barely had the time to say goodbye to my daughter before the next contraction came along. We got to hospital at 4.15a.m. and I had to go on all fours outside the hospital while we waited to be let in, my husband putting pressure on my back while I breathed through it. Upon my arrival I had decided to have a vaginal examination and I was grateful to hear I was already eight centimetres dilated…but annoyed that they wouldn't let me in the bath. I guess they thought I was going to be quite quick as the midwives phoned my obstetrician at this time.

I only spent an hour in the shower (the hose on my abdomen and the shower falling on my back) before I had to come back to the bed to start pushing. All had gone so well and so fast up to this point, my husband and I were elated and thinking 'this isn't so bad'. However, at this point I was in full transition and needed gas, so I went on all fours on the bed. This is when the labour went into slow motion. I really wanted to push but my waters hadn't broken and this seemed to stall my progress. I know now that even though I thought I had let go of the fear attached to my first labour, I still had fear connected to pushing the baby out, having had intervention the first time. I kept saying again and again, 'I can't do this on my own', and the midwife responded with, 'Yes you can, you are in control.' But the negative thoughts just kept creeping back after I went into transition and I couldn't stop them.

I kept thinking, 'What if he's stuck and I am doing all this work for nothing, and I have to have a Caesarean?' This thought had been planted by my obstetrician over the previous weeks, telling me frequently how big this baby was and, 'Don't you think you should have a Caesarean and avoid complications?' I had told him that I wanted to wait and see what happens, as no one could know how big he was going to be. However, my strength had deserted me while in full labour and I began to weaken, and I know that this made the pushing much harder and longer than it needed to be. Despite this, the only intervention I needed was for my waters to be broken, and I pushed Charlie Jack out at 7.06a.m., after having been at the hospital for only two hours! The midwife told me later that he had had his little fist on his cheek, and that had made it difficult for him to come through my birth canal, NOT his size, which was seven pounds twelve ounces, an average-size baby to say the least.

So, even though I agree that all birth experiences are individual, my experience shows that what you really need is to have the right kind of emotional and mental preparation. Not allowing negative or self-doubting thoughts to take over is equally as important. Lastly, really trust yourself and your own body and you can achieve an amazing birth experience.

Sean And Sally's Birth Journey

The old adage is true. Go on holiday, relax and you'll come back pregnant. Sean and I were in the last eight weeks of our six-month world tour when I discovered I was pregnant. We bought the test on my twenty-eighth birthday in Oxford, England. After dinner and a movie we sat in a beautiful bed-and-breakfast in shock. Although we wanted children, we thought I would fall pregnant after our holiday. Needless to say, we were overjoyed. We continued travelling but came home a couple of weeks early. Our bank balance was suffering and so was I with morning sickness. Sickness that lasted all day and all night.

It was great to be back in Australia after being away for six months. Travelling really showed us we were lucky to live here. With no money it was straight back to work for the both of us. Not so easy when one is vomiting all the time! Luckily I only had to endure that for sixteen weeks.

Through an old work colleague, I learned there were aqua-aerobic classes for pregnancy at my local swimming pool. My first lesson was during my fourteenth week of pregnancy and although I still felt very average, the class lifted my spirits and made me feel great. It was the relaxation, being towed around the pool by another person, that had me hooked. In fact this was the first time I had actually relaxed since Sean and I had returned from overseas.

At the classes run by Gaby I found out that she also ran ongoing Active Birth classes, which I started to attend. They opened my eyes to a whole new world in which I met other women who, like me, wanted to know about birth and had little idea of what to expect. Even though I was myself a nurse and I had attended many births previously, you really do see the birth process through different eyes when you are the one who is pregnant. Not only did I make some wonderful friends, but I found someone I could trust to support me in bringing my baby into the world in a loving, supportive way.

As my tummy began to swell, I started to think about my birthing options, and Sean and I made the decision to have Gaby as our doula. We thought it would be helpful to have guidance through such a positive life-changing experience and really gave our thoughts lots of time and attention. I am a good organiser and wanted to be really well-prepared for the birth-day and not just leave it to the mentality of 'We'll just see what happens on the day'. I loved being pregnant and loved the way I looked and felt. I have never been one to show off my body but I believed I looked fantastic and was happy to show off my belly to anyone who wanted to see it.

As the birth-day drew nearer I kept in close contact with Gaby, who allayed so many of my fears. Fears of becoming a parent, fear of birth and just the feeling of being plain scared.

I had experienced a couple of antepartum bleeds, which fortunately didn't amount to anything – in fact I found out through talking to lots of other women that they are quite common. On this particular day I thought I was having another one, however this turned out to be my 'show'.

On 26 August I awoke at 6 a.m. after a rather unsettled night, to empty my bladder, and experienced my first contraction. So that is what they feel like, I was thinking, and I felt so excited. After hurrying back to the bedroom to tell my partner, I then asked him to open the curtains so we could watch the sun come up together. It was so beautiful being able to experience this moment with just the two of us knowing that on this day we were going to have our baby.

The contractions were three minutes apart from the beginning. I was handling them really well. So well, in fact, that when Gaby arrived at 9a.m., I said to her, 'This feels really great, bring it on!' With that Gaby smiled with an amused look on her face. Gaby was pleased to hear that I was so accepting and enthusiastic about the contractions and later commented to me how wonderful it was to hear a woman talk like this prior to going into more established labour.

Soon after, I was moving about the house from station to station. I had a great position on our bed, leaning over the beanbag and pillows, then I moved to the shower, followed by the bath, then onto the fitball in the lounge. It was a happening thing. I moved between these stations in between the contractions, really utilising what each station and position had to offer me. This really helped to pass the time and to cope with the intensity. Having Sean and Gaby at my side also made a huge difference as I felt so supported and strong.

By about 2p.m. we decided it was time to go to the hospital. I was petrified I would have contractions in the car on the way to hospital and no one would be able to assist me in any way. I feel that because of this fear I stopped my labour temporarily on the way to hospital, as I did not have one single contraction in the time it took to get there. Getting out of the car and into the hospital was a whole other matter. As soon as I stepped foot outside of the car I had three contractions in a row, right in front of a group of visitors to the hospital. They disbanded in various directions and disappeared as soon as they could, thank goodness.

It was a long walk to the labour ward as I had to stop many

times and lean on Sean, the wall or Gaby to get through the intensity, as they were coming on thick and fast at this point. At this stage I felt the need to start using the visualisations and breathing Gaby had taught me and this really helped me to keep myself and the contractions under control.

The next few hours went past in a blur. I do remember having an internal examination just prior to getting in the shower. An internal was something I really did not want to have, so I had one but requested that I not be told how dilated I was. Thankfully the midwife did not tell me. The next day I actually found out that I was four centimetres at that stage, but it took me less than four hours from then to have my baby.

I found myself giving birth on a mattress that was on the floor, leaning over a beanbag with pillows on top. It was funny really, as I had always pictured myself semi squatting on the floor, but when the time came this felt just right. With every contraction Sean and Gaby would apply pressure and lots of it to my lower back, which felt fantastic at the time. As the baby came down and started to stretch my perineum I requested a hot flannel on there, which felt wonderful and really took the sting away. I felt like I was screaming at this time but Sean tells me I was reasonably quiet, all things considered.

At one point an anaesthetist accidentally walked into our room, and Gaby and Sean called out, 'I think you have the wrong room, we don't need you here', and all I was thinking to myself was, 'Come back, come back, I need you.' In the next moment I was telling myself, 'No I don't, I'm a strong woman having a baby now.' It was like having an angel on one shoulder telling me I can do it and the devil on the other shoulder trying to convince me to have an epidural. The angel triumphed, as it was nearly all over and I was starting to push my baby out of my body.

After just thirty minutes of pushing with Gaby's guidance and support I was able to push my beautiful baby out and into the waiting hands of Sean and the midwife. They then slowly passed my baby through my legs, where I held him skin to skin on my chest. I then turned around slowly and sat down so that Sean and I could discover the sex of our baby.

And there he was. Dark blue eyes blinking, and staring up at me. His hair darker than I had anticipated, glistening in the light. His perfect hands clasped together. His body moist and soft. Wow, what a moment.

I tried him on my breast but he was more content to be cuddled. I was awash with emotion. Love, glorious love. Amazement. How could two people create this perfect little angel? Thankfulness – he and I were both healthy. Exhaustion – labour is tough, no doubt about it, but you live to tell the story over and over of how wonderful it is – that, I guess, is the irony.

This is the beginning. We knew having a baby would change us forever and it has, for the better. For this reason it was so important to have our baby in a calm, loving and unobtrusive environment. We wanted to start our new life together in the best possible way. We are eternally grateful that our dream and wishes were granted.

A Birth Story About Jack

I was thirty-nine when I gave birth to Jack, who is my first and only child. The journey through my pregnancy was just as big as the birthing experience itself as I struggled to come to terms with what impending motherhood meant for me. My background is exercise physiology, then more recently horse training and riding instruction. When I realised I was pregnant we were halfway through building a substantial house (my husband Mike is a builder) and my show-jumping and dressage riding was in full swing. While I had never discarded the thought of having a baby, I had not actively sought one either.

At about the four-month mark I became very emotional about my identity and self-esteem, which were taking a severe dive. I felt I was dropping into a deep chasm of worthlessness, losing my personal identity and my standing in the horse fraternity. All this was based on a belief that if I wasn't out there achieving academically or physically (being a sporting hero) I really was just a 'nothing' in society. The dysfunctional belief I had is that anyone can be a 'breeding female'. I won't delve into where these beliefs came from, but they were picked up during my childhood and were having a very powerful destabilising influence. It took a number of counselling sessions and a weekend workshop of cathartic release to finally bring up, deal with and disempower these dysfunctional ideas.

Nearing the birth I had participated in Gaby's birthing education sessions. These were highly beneficial and far more informative than the hospital-based course. I had chosen Gaby as my doula as she is a close friend and well-versed in birthing! I had also assisted in the birth of her third child, for whom I am the godmother. Also, with my knowledge of exercise physiology, I understood and practised the technique of PNF stretching (Proprioceptive Neuromuscular Facilitation) of the perineum.

The perineum is a muscle just like any other muscle, so it will respond to specific stretching exercises. I used this technique three times a week over the final six weeks of the pregnancy and had no tearing at all. Gaby even commented at the birth that I had the most 'stretchy' perineum she had seen. I believe this technique should be taught in all prenatal classes as it has a very powerful effect by helping the perineum release during birth.

My due date was 28 September, and as this date came and went panic set in, as I was desperate to avoid induction. 'D Day' was to be Thursday 9 October. On the night of 6 October I had a false labour (poor Gaby drove all the way out to Wandi, twenty minutes south of Perth, WA, at midnight, only to have things grind to a halt). This really triggered a depression, and I banned all talk of pregnancy, babies, etc., as I had had enough. I refused to take phone calls from anyone and would get very annoyed when someone did manage to catch me.

I was now into gulping castor oil, jogging around the block (both were equally as uncomfortable) and self-stimulation to try to bring it along. Finally I listened to my intuition and sought the help of a spiritual friend who performed an attunement with me. I cried in this session as I connected with my baby in a way which he was needing but I had been denying. He also communicated to me his fear about the pain of birthing. I had never thought to see things from his angle before, and this realisation was very moving for me.

Well, twenty-four hours later on the night before 'D Day' I was finally in labour. At 10p.m. I felt a little weird and the waters broke with a trickle. I quietly went downstairs so as not to involve Mike. I laboured away for three hours, timing the contractions until I knew we had to start making a move to the Family Birthing Centre. The contractions were becoming moderately painful by the time I called to Mike, who immediately flew into panic. I hadn't contemplated that keeping his hormones down was going to be on my list of duties in birthing! We called Gaby and she arrived around 1.30a.m. She suggested staying at home for a while longer just to make sure I was heading into full labour, but I said, 'No, we go right now', as I felt the contractions were becoming significantly stronger.

At 3a.m. we arrived at the centre. An internal found I was only two centimetres – I thought to myself, 'Heck, is that all, for all this work I am doing!' Thank goodness the midwife didn't tell me the baby was also posterior or I would have given up. Lying on my back for the internals was agony. My body shook uncontrollably and caused the contractions to get stronger afterwards. Looking back I should not have had the internals as I felt they aggravated the intensity of the contractions and gave me an anterior lip, which ultimately made birthing more difficult, as I had to breathe on contractions hard and not bear down on this swelling tissue. Easier said than done!

At the five-hour mark I was hitting the wall with intense contractions and feeling that things were going nowhere – only four centimetres dilated! I cried out that I wanted to quit, that I was allowed to quit! I wanted to give up and have the epidural. The midwife suggested I try gas, which I choked on and threw the mouthpiece down onto the floor. Eventually the midwives offered me a shot of pethidine, which gave me three hours of wonderful bliss in the bath where I slept in between contractions.

As the pethidine effects started to wear off and the contractions returned in their full intensity, it was back to work for the home run. I walked between contractions and sat on the loo during them. This helped a lot as you give yourself permission to really open up and not be embarrassed at the consequences. After having had so much castor oil my bowels were in full swing. Trying to hold it in is not good when you need to open up for the baby to come down.

At the fourteen hours mark I was eight centimetres and nothing was happening apart from the very strong contractions, which made me grip onto my husband and cry out my stress! At this time I was starting to hit the wall, so I decided I wanted to transfer up to the main part of the hospital so I could have an epidural.

After a spinal block, which is a mild form of epidural, was put into my back I slept a little and rested my tired body. However, before long I was fully awake and aware of the need to push. As the spinal wore off the need to push increased. After fifteen hours of labour I got down off the bed and onto the floor to birth my baby with the full sensation of what I needed to do. My son Jack slid into the world in a calm and peaceful way.

Would I do it all again the same way? Definitely. The experience of a natural birth is something I will hold dear forever.

I must say I was in awe of my husband for keeping so mentally present during the whole labour. I never knew he had it in him! Knowing when to be quiet and sensitive and then when to grip me like heck as a support during the toughest times. Having a trusted and competent support team is essential to a good birthing experience.

After twenty-four hours we were ready to bring Jack home. We feel truly blessed with the birth of our beautiful little boy. He has made our lives so complete.

Matthew's Birth Story – A Home Water-Birth

I was woken at 7a.m. with an almighty contraction. I'd had a feeling the night before that it was just about time, so I was well prepared. I was planning a homebirth as I'd had previous hospital and Birth Centre births. This time I preferred to stay at home in my own environment with my husband Brett and our two other children, Jarrod and Melanie.

I was planning a water birth, so I had the tub set up ready in the lounge room, where I could see out into the garden. I had all my special things arranged in the room – my picture of the Madonna, some fresh flowers, crystals, oil burner with all my oils ready, CD player and music (relaxation and belly-dancing music) and family photo. I had my flower and gem essences ready to take and my aromatherapy massage blend all set to go.

At 8.15 a.m. I rang my midwife, Kate, to let her know I was in labour. I hadn't had a show at this point and my membranes were still intact, but I felt like things were moving along quite quickly. I was contracting every two to three minutes. I also rang my parents, who were my support team. Mum had been my doula for the previous two births and Dad had been at the first, but missed the second. They always proved to be a wonderful help with support for Brett and myself and the children.

Once I'd called everyone the contractions seemed to slow down to five to ten minutes apart. I decided to have a shower and eat some breakfast just in case it turned out to be a long day after all. Brett cooked up a big pot of porridge and we all sat down to eat. I managed to get through with only a couple of contractions and it felt like labour was fizzling out.

It was about ten o'clock before anyone arrived, as Dad had to be called back home from the golf course and Kate had to drive across to the other side of town to pick up all her equipment.

There was a knock on the door. I answered it to find Mum and Dad expecting to see me in full-on labour. I was feeling like a bit of a fake at this point. Once they were in and settled I got a couple of whopper contractions which took me completely by surprise. But when they were finished I felt bright and alert.

It wasn't until Kate arrived at 10.45 a.m. that it really started happening! I had the most full-on, sharp, bottom-piercing contractions that I've ever experienced. It felt like I was sitting on a spear! Now I was desperate to go to the toilet (as a midwife myself, I know this is a sign of second stage – but I had to go!). I was sitting on the toilet feeling the head looming down and all I could hear was Kate saying, 'Get off the toilet, Faye, you're having your baby.'

It was lucky that Brett had taken charge of getting the tub ready for me, because we made a cross-legged manoeuvre for it in between contractions. I climbed into it with great relief, just in time for the head to start emerging. I had the pleasure and the honour of guiding my son's head out into the warm water. Matthew Joseph Read was born at 11.18 a.m. (just thirty-three minutes after Kate's arrival) on 5 July 1995.

The first thing Matthew saw was a sea of faces peering in at him from the edge of the tub. There was Mum and Dad, his brother Jarrod, sister Melanie, Gran and Granddad and Kate. He floated around for a while, taking it all in before settling into me for his first breastfeed while we snuggled together in the warm tub.

After about half an hour we decided to get out of the tub for the delivery of the placenta, which came away nicely and all together. I cut the cord for Matthew, which seemed very symbolic. Later we showed the inquisitive kids what it was and how it worked. They were rather fascinated. We then wrapped Matthew up all nice and warm while I went off to have a shower. The birth took place on a Wednesday, and as this is the day that my family usually gets together we phoned my two sisters and invited them to come over and have 'family day' at our house. They both arrived soon after, loaded up with food and drinks for lunch. We all sat down together to celebrate the wonderful event with a mandatory glass of champagne. When I came down from my 'high', I decided to slip upstairs and have a sleep with my new baby. The others crept out quietly a little later on.

About a week later we had a private 'naming ceremony' in our backyard with those present on the birthday, and then we planted the placenta under a special rose bush that we had bought for the occasion.

I had the most wonderful birth experience that I could ever have hoped for. I thank my wonderful family and midwife for all their fantastic support.

A Wonderful Birth Experience

Excited at the prospect of the birth of my first baby, I wanted to do everything possible to make it a safe and wonderful experience. I asked Gaby to assist me at the birth, as my partner, David, is extremely squeamish and didn't feel up to being present during the entire birth. Also, we had moved to Western Australia only a few months before the baby was due and I didn't have anyone else to be with me. As I was thirty-six at the time I also felt quite anxious about the possibility of things going wrong and wanted someone there with Gaby's experience.

Gaby and I had a few long talks about my birth plan. I told her I wanted a natural birth – I hated the idea of having a needle put into my spine, and didn't want to interfere with the birth process – knowing that it would make further intervention more likely.

My contractions started at about 9.30 p.m. with mild crampy pains. By about 12 p.m. the pains were getting a bit more intense, but I still wasn't quite sure if I was in labour. I began timing the pains and realised they were five minutes apart. About an hour later I had a show and the pains were quite gripping, so I woke David and told him the baby was on its way. We rang the maternity hospital and the nurse I spoke to suggested I take a Panadol and go back to bed. I don't think so! David made me a cup of tea and I slowly got my bag together and then decided to go in to the hospital. When we got there they put us in a little room with two beds and David tried to get some more sleep. I lay down but when each contraction came I had to stand up and pace the floor.

After a short while Gaby arrived and David decided to drive home to drop off the dog (she had come with us to the hospital and was waiting in the car). To be honest I was glad to see him relieved of his duty – he obviously felt a bit out of place and I really only wanted to be among women who understood the birth process. It was a big relief to have Gaby there, who immediately set up some pillows on the bed and gave me a fitball to sit on. I think I stayed in this position for quite a while, and just put my head into the pillow during each contraction, while Gaby massaged a special essential oil into my back. After a while it felt time for a change and Gaby showed me another position, leaning against the wall with my arms above my head. That was surprisingly comfortable and I had all my other contractions in that position.

I breathed through each contraction and that allowed me to focus on something else rather than the pain. When the pain increased, Gaby and I went to the shower and she held the hose over my back or my tummy for each contraction. I stayed in the shower for what seemed like a long time, until eventually I felt a bit waterlogged and we went back to my room, which smelt beautiful due to the massage oil. Every now and then the midwife came in to see how things were going. Gaby let her know that I didn't want to have an internal examination until it was really necessary and that I had chosen not to have pain relief (unless it was also really necessary).

After changing to the standing position for my contractions, my pains came on more intensely and more frequently. I sometimes had a shorter contraction (with no peak to it) followed by another shorter one about two minutes later. When things got hard to bear, Gaby and I went to the shower again. Later, when we got back in the room, I started feeling a bit anxious about how much longer the labour would take. Gaby asked me to visualise the size of my cervix and I had a really clear image of a circle with a diameter of about 71.5 centimetres. More time passed, with me standing against the wall, breathing into each contraction (they were pretty intense at this stage) and Gaby massaging my back. David came in at one point after returning to the hospital and wished me well before going off to the waiting room.

One hour later, I started to feel anxious again and worried about how much longer the labour would take. Gaby asked me to do another visualisation and this time the circle was about 91.5 centimetres in diameter. Shortly afterward there was a change of shift among the nursing staff and a new midwife came in to introduce herself. She said she would like to do an internal soon as they weren't sure that I was in established labour – this wasn't what I wanted to hear! The midwife decided to give me more time and about half an hour later as I was getting ready for another contraction I heard a loud splat as my waters broke onto the floor.

The feeling of the contractions changed – I could now feel the bulk of the baby in my pelvis. The midwife came in and asked to check the baby's heartbeat as she said there was a small amount of meconium in the amniotic fluid. The heartbeat on the monitor was strong and steady and I felt a huge relief knowing that the baby was doing well through all this. Gaby was wonderfully supportive and calm and kept talking to me in a gentle, soft voice. Still I felt anxious and later Gaby told me I was probably in transition at this stage. I told Gaby I would agree to an internal but that I only wanted to hear the results if they were good.

As the nurse put on her gloves I had another contraction and had to jump up off the bed, there was no way I could cope with a contraction lying on my back.

After the internal Gaby and the nurse said it was time to go to the birthing room (later Gaby told me I was ten centimetres dilated and the head was two centimetres through – so much for not reaching established labour!). Once there, I had about two more contractions against the wall and then they set up pillows on the birthing bed for me to lean against. During contractions I now felt an urge to push and at the same time open my mouth wide and let out noise (David tells me it was VERY LOUD). I think I expected the baby to pop out pretty quickly and as it took a while I had to ask if the baby was stuck. I was told it wasn't and after twenty minutes out it came. I think I slumped forward onto the pillows until I heard the baby cry – I turned around and there was my little baby girl. I certainly had my wonderful experience, and I felt so grateful for Gaby's presence, which was like having an angel watching over me, and finally David and I got to meet our little miracle!

Births Of William And Ella

Monday 15 April 2002

No matter how many books you read or how many birthing classes you attend, nothing really adequately prepares you for your first birthing experience.

Being aware of alternative procedures prior to the birth of my baby boy, in addition to the standardised hospital procedures, gave me the confidence to arrive at the hospital armed with viable options. Having confidence is especially important to me, and going into an experience for the first time can be daunting, so having an alternative birthing plan made it less so.

I woke at 3a.m. with some discomfort. We had open backstairs at the time and I managed to ease some of the discomfort by stretching my arms to a stair and rocking backwards and forwards on my fitball. After having some breakfast we arrived at the hospital at around 10a.m. where I was given an immediate internal. I was only one centimetre dilated so it was a case of just trying to remain as comfortable as possible using the shower, stretching and massage.

At noon I was beginning to feel quite tired, my waters had only just broken and the contractions were steady at around five minutes apart. At 12.30p.m. I was given another internal and was told that I was now four centimetres dilated. At this stage I was having difficulty coping with the pain and in hindsight I probably should have checked out the gas and air as a source of pain relief instead of opting for an epidural.

At 1.30p.m. the epidural was administered and within twenty minutes all pain had gone and so all I could feel was the painless tightening with each contraction. At 4.30p.m. my skin felt itchy all over, I'm not sure if this was a combination of the hot shower and the epidural. By 5.30p.m. I was given a drip to help speed up my contractions. This had an immediate effect on the strength and frequency of my contractions, prompting the mid-wife to suggest that I lie on the bed to relieve the pressure of the contractions and to speed up the baby's heart rate as it was very slow.

At 6.30p.m. I asked for a top-up of the epidural. I'd become used to no pain for over five hours, so as the initial epidural wore off painful contractions started to come on very quickly, becoming too much to handle, as I was by now extremely tired and feeling quite exhausted. In hindsight, once again I should have taken this opportunity to try gas and air because I'm convinced that the top-up of the epidural slowed the birth down again.

At 8.40p.m. I was fully dilated, but I still could not experience the contractions to their full effect and had to rely on the midwife telling me when to push. On the bed I was in a half sitting, half lying position, with my knees bent and my legs held by my partner and my sister. This position does not assist the birth of a baby whatsoever, but because of the epidural and subsequent lack of sensation in my legs, it was impossible for me to get into my planned position of being on all fours and offer my baby a much better angle for delivery.

At 11.13p.m., some twenty-odd hours after hanging from my stairs, I finally gave birth to a beautiful baby boy weighing a healthy seven pounds fifteen ounces. The euphoria was wonderful, along with the fabulous endorphins racing through my body – the whole conception of birth is an absolute miracle. New life is beyond written or spoken words. However, I can't help feeling that my miracle was only part of the true journey of childbirth because of the effect the epidural had, not only on myself, but also on my baby's first few hours.

Saturday 1 November 2003

The story continues with the birth of Ella, my second baby. During the afternoon I'd taken a long walk to try and get things started. I was far more composed with this pregnancy and I felt like I was much more in control. The fear of entering the unknown, mixed with all the horror stories that certain people feel they have to tell you, as was the case with my first birth, were not in evidence this time around. I knew that this time I would be more positive and resist the temptation of complete pain relief and give myself, and my baby, a far better birthing experience than before.

At around 7.30p.m. I started to feel a little nauseous and physically tired so decided to have a warm bath and try to relax. As soon as I got into the bath contractions started immediately. However, I was determined to stay in the bath and enjoy this experience, plus I didn't want to spend hours at the hospital again. After ten minutes I couldn't remain lying in the bath, as things were happening very quickly and it all took me rather by surprise. My husband checked the duration and frequency of the contractions and we were both quite shocked and very excited once we discovered that they were only three minutes apart and lasting around a minute.

Once my Mum arrived to look after William, we set off in the car to the hospital, which is only a twenty-minute drive away. I had to lift myself from the car seat as I could feel the baby's head bearing down. I honestly thought at this stage that I was going to give birth in the car. The time was now 9.10 p.m., and once inside the hospital and positioned on all fours on the bed, the midwife informed me that I was fully dilated. I was given the option of gas and air for my pain relief, which was fantastic. I was in complete control, managing the breathing, totally focused and being able to understand and feel my baby's journey into the world. It was an incredible experience as I felt so in touch with my baby, as we worked together in the most beautiful way possible.

Ella came into the world naturally at 10.10 p.m., with no tear and me being on all fours just like I had imagined I would have been. This time around I felt so mentally and physically prepared and so happy. I created a much more positive birth experience for the both of us.

I can't fully explain how different the two births were. Obviously both were fantastic experiences, with a beautiful gift of life at the end. However, given the chance again, I would choose my second birthing experience over the first without doubt, as I was the one in control, yet surrendering at the same time.

Soren's Breech Vbac Birth

On 12 September 2004 I gave birth to my son Soren by vaginal breech birth. His birth has captured the imagination of many people, since it was a vaginal birth after a previous Caesarean (VBAC) and a spontaneous vaginal breech birth. For me, I was simply doing what my body told me I had to do on the day.

I am ecstatic at the birth and the outcome, although nothing went according to plan! I give full credit to my support team (husband Mick and private midwife) and the hospital staff (midwife and obstetrician) who attended me on the day – I couldn't have done it without them.

So what happened?

The story of Soren's birth starts about four years earlier with the birth of my first child, a daughter, Tessa, on 1 September 2000. I was very ill with a liver problem (obstetric cholestasis) in the third trimester of my pregnancy with her and she was presenting breech, so at thirty-seven weeks she was born by Caesarean section. We were thrilled to have our lovely daughter and my health improved immediately. However, my recovery from the Caesarean section was long, slow and painful and it took months to establish breastfeeding. Now Tessa is a delightful, happy, healthy four-year-old.

When we decided to try for a second child, I knew I really wanted to avoid getting obstetric cholestasis again if I could, and I also wanted to birth vaginally rather than by Caesarean section. After more than a year of pre-conception care under the guidance of a naturopath, we were brimming with health and I became pregnant a second time.

I chose a private obstetrician who was prepared to support me for a VBAC. He advised that I had a ninety per cent chance of the obstetric cholestasis recurring, but was unable to suggest any preventative measures.

I had been advised that a knowledgeable support person such as a doula or midwife was important for a VBAC, so I also engaged a private midwife. She cared for and supported me throughout the pregnancy and was the best thing that ever happened to me. I also kept working with the naturopath to optimise my liver function through herbs, diet and reflexology. I was very fit and healthy throughout the pregnancy. No signs of obstetric cholestasis.

My broad plan for the birth was to labour at home and then birth in hospital. Towards the end of the pregnancy I even started to consider the possibility of a homebirth.

I put a lot of effort into preparing myself for the birth. In fact, I gave up all notions of working that year in favour of birth preparation. As well as preparing my body – walking, swimming, yoga – I put most effort into preparing my mind! I read widely, and saw for the first time that birth was not all about pain and fear, and that someone like me – conservative, averse to pain, not overly maternal – could have a 'good birth'. It was a revelation, and at the same time very challenging – could I actually do it? I talked to women, meditated, went to birth preparation classes, sought counselling to deal with some 'old baggage', and went over and over the birth scenario with my midwife.

At thirty-five weeks the preparation stopped and our thoughts went on a tangent – the baby was laying breech. The next four weeks were a time of great stress as we tried everything in the book to encourage the baby to turn – lying upside down on an angled plank, crawling on all fours, handstands in the swimming pool, homeopathics, pressure on the little toes, moxa sticks, acupuncture, energy work and visualisation – all to no avail. At thirty-nine weeks the obstetrician attempted to turn the baby by external cephalic version (ECV) but it was not successful. The baby did not want to turn. At this point I decided not to try anything further to turn the baby – it clearly did not want to be head-down!

Being pregnant with a breech baby is a rather lonely road. I was preoccupied with dealing with the breech situation, while the other pregnant women I met were happily getting on with their birth preparation. We had nothing in common at that time. I felt very alone, especially when I realised that the decision about what to do was entirely mine. After the ECV, even though unsuccessful, it was a great relief to move forward, to get on with the business of having a baby rather than focusing on the breech. Of course, my birth options had rather narrowed! A homebirth was out of the question.

The obstetrician was quite specific: the birth would be by Caesarean section; a vaginal birth was not an option. He agreed to allow me to go into labour and then do the Caesarean section, so at least the timing of the birth would be natural, if not the birth itself. I was pleased that at least my baby would be setting the birth agenda. We planned to birth at a local hospital.

My midwife's thinking was not limited to a Caesarean section, however. She often advised me that a vaginal birth of a breech baby would be possible at King Edward Memorial Hospital (KEMH) if I wanted it, and if we exercised our rights and strongly insisted on it with hospital staff. I could not imagine being able to labour effectively if I was in an adversarial situation with hospital staff over my birthing choices, so I was not prepared to pursue the vaginal birth option any further. I agreed to the Caesarean section, with the arrangement being that I'd labour at home for a few hours before coming to hospital.

Four days after my baby's due date was a Saturday. I woke up feeling different; something was imminent. I had a near-constant hard stomach with Braxton-Hicks contractions. The day and evening passed uneventfully – Mick finished the house project he was working on and we put Tessa to bed. I was still feeling 'different' but had nothing to report when we went to bed at 11.30 p.m.

Labour started immediately. The contractions were about fifteen minutes apart and I was able to breathe comfortably through them while lying in bed. Over the next four hours the contractions gradually got closer and more intense. I stayed in bed but was not able to sleep at all. At 4 a.m. on Sunday morning I was no longer comfortable in bed and I went downstairs. I dressed and lit a candle. Outside it was a beautiful clear starry night. I pottered around putting the last few things in my hospital bag. I leant on my kitchen bench for each contraction and was then able to continue my chores. I had to go to the toilet between each contraction.

At 4.30 a.m. contractions were five to six minutes apart and intense and I had a bloody show. I woke Mick and told him it was time to call our midwife. Mick started to massage my back with each contraction. My contractions were intense and hard work, but I would not say painful.

Our midwife arrived shortly after our call. I laboured on; I felt I was handling the contractions without distress and I was relaxed and able to chat in between. In fact part of me wondered if this was the real thing! At 6 a.m., just before Mum and Dad arrived to mind Tessa, a vaginal examination showed that I was six centimetres dilated. I was elated and amazed, as it had been relatively easy to that point. Obviously we would have to get going to hospital pretty soon for the Caesarean section.

Our midwife phoned the obstetrician to fill him in. He reiterated that he would not support a vaginal birth. Our midwife reminded me of my options: we could go off to the local hospital for the Caesarean section as planned or we could still change our minds and go to KEMH for a vaginal birth. A decision was required, and soon! It was down to me! Mick would support whatever I decided. For the first time I entertained the idea of a vaginal breech birth (VBAC). I was well progressed in labour and handling it well. I knew about the risks – I'd done my homework. I thought of coming home a few hours later with my baby or a few days later with a painful wound and my baby. Outside it was a beautiful spring morning.

For once in my life my brain was not weighing up pros and cons. Rather, I just knew what had to be done. It's hard to explain, but this baby had to be birthed vaginally. I felt this in my body very strongly. So I made the call. We would go to KEMH for a vaginal breech birth.

Our midwife was on the phone again, advising the obstetrician that his services were longer required and letting KEMH know that we were on our way. Then we literally flew to KEMH–

Fremantle to Subiaco in twelve minutes – the fastest trip of our lives. Thank goodness it was 7 a.m. on a Sunday.

Sitting in the car was painful. It felt like I was sitting on the baby. On arrival at KEMH I was offered a wheelchair but couldn't bear the idea of sitting down. So I walked to the labour ward; everybody jumped when my waters broke en route!

At the labour ward we met our delightful hospital midwife, who was more than willing to help me birth my breech baby. She had organised a mobile foetal heart monitor so I could move and birth standing up. Baby was fine. I was now fully dilated with a slight lip, so I panted through a couple of contractions while we waited for the lip to go and for the consultant obstetrician to start her shift.

The consultant obstetrician was warm and kind and she very calmly advised me of the risks of proceeding with the breech VBAC, including that the baby could die. She offered me a Caesarean section even at that late stage. (I noted that no one outlined any risks of a Caesarean section to me!) She then very kindly offered me encouragement in what I was doing and said that she thought things were proceeding well. She also told me she was experienced with breech births. What more could I want in the way of support? It was wonderful. I restated my desire to birth vaginally. After that, I was down to business.

I was birthing standing up, hanging around Mick's neck to bear down. It was amusing to glance down and see the consultant and midwives crouching awkwardly on the floor, looking up at my nether regions! I took a while to get the hang of pushing. The baby's bottom was in view, but not out yet. After a while our private midwife could see that an episiotomy was looming so she told me to give it my all. I held my breath and pushed with all my might. At last the bottom was born. The rest of the body, the limbs and then the head followed quickly, with only minor assistance – the consultant's finger inserted in the baby's mouth to pull the jaw down and head forward. There was no time to get onto the bed to birth the head as the consultant had wished – I heard her ask for a cloth to catch the baby, and he was out!

After four hours of established labour and an hour of pushing, my breech boy was in my arms, on my breast, us both in a heap on the floor. I could not believe that the birth was over, that he was with us, that all was well. I was filled with wonder and gratitude. It was 9 a.m. Our four-year-old Tessa came to join us and meet her brother at lunchtime. We went home at 3 p.m. And named him Soren.

Afterwards, I realised just how wonderful our private midwife had been for us. She made all the phone calls to the original obstetrician and hospital and to KEMH, shielding us from the flak that I'm sure was flying. She advised the hospital staff of the wishes I'd expressed in my birth plan (and which, in all the hurly-burly, I'd forgotten to mention), including my desire to birth standing up and my wish to birth the placenta naturally, without an injection. She stated my wishes and they were respected. I did not have to argue my case. And then her presence and care made it possible for us to go home the same day. She endured our freezing house while I laboured and did not express alarm at travelling at 120 kilometres an hour through suburban streets to hospital!

The next day, when I reflected on my decision to go for a vaginal birth, I was shocked. Seriously shocked. When I looked at the situation from my rational (not birthing) perspective, I could not believe I'd taken the risk of a vaginal birth. Just one day later, I was no longer driven by instincts, I was back inside my head.

I feel blessed to have a beautiful, healthy son and I'm so grateful for the journey and the experience that my pregnancy and Soren's birth have been.

27
Estelle's Epilogue

It is twenty-three years since the first baby was born in my bath-tub. The mother, the midwife and I were committed to the process of using water as a birthing tool, in light of the information received from Dr Michel Odent and Igor Charkovsky that it was perfectly safe.

There were less than one hundred water-born babies worldwide at that time, 1982. Today there are thousands of mothers and babies who have used water to promote a safe, gentle, non-intrusive birth. In Great Britain in 1994 the research proving safety allowed the British Government to legislate to enable women in the UK to choose water as a birthing option in all hospitals, even on their national health scheme. The general resistance from medical professionals has largely been in America, Australia and other countries, where birth has become a major medical procedure, with evidence to question the outcomes.

As a pioneer of water birth, my issue is that an expectant mother must have as much information as possible to help her make an informed choice, be it in a bed, a bath, at home or hospital. Then she should be totally supported in her choice. Every

A labour of love

birth is a miracle and unique; most women, given the appropriate support, can create new life and bring it into the world just as they were designed by nature to do.

Gaby is a mother of three water-born babies, a birth educator using water for prenatal purposes, and also the teacher of aquatics to new babies and their parents. Her experience plus her training makes her an excellent authority on the subject. This book is a brilliant contribution of practical and experiental knowledge to those seeking valid information about the process. As a mother and grandmother, and a witness to water births in many countries over the last twenty-three years, it is my opinion that what a woman needs when giving birth is the experience of another woman. You do not need a doctor to make a baby, and it follows that unless there are serious reasons, you do not need a doctor to 'deliver' a newborn. In fact it is a labour of love, and the baby a gift of that love, and the father should be the one who catches the gift of love returned.

This book holds authentic and valuable information and should be read by anyone planning to have or be involved in a water birth.

Estelle Myers
MA App. Sc, Hon. PhD

Acknowledgements

A sincere thank you to:

Liz Stubbs, mother of four, editor extraordinaire, who gave tirelessly to reading, re-reading and editing my manuscripts for this book. I appreciate every moment of your time and hard work in getting this book into some sort of shape – thank you from the core of my soul.

Tracy Duff who did the most remarkable job typesetting my initial self-published book and creating my labour of love image. They say, in small things big things grow, well they, who ever they are, were right. The huge effort, creatively, has been fantastic and something I will never forget. Thank you for all that you have done for me. I will be forever greatful.

Cathy Cooksey who designed the graphic images for the book. Amid having your own baby you still had the time to complete the artistic images for me. Thank you for your multi- tasking skills.

Susan Maushart for your words of wisdom, and encouragement. I said to you once, 'I am not a writer, but if you would be willing to read my manuscripts I would be thrilled'. You replied, 'Gaby no one is a true writer until they have got all of their thoughts down onto the paper, and played around with the ideas, so don't let that stand in your way'. I listened, and here it is!

All of the wonderful women/couples whom I have had the privilege to doula for. Each and every one of you taught me more than you will ever know, enabling me to write this book based on what I observed and learnt. I am very humbled and honored to have been a part of something so incredible.

All the wonderful women attending my aquatic classes at the Fremantle Leisure Centre who listen to my stories, and open their hearts to share theirs, in an honest environment. The sharing made a huge difference in the lives of many who have attended over the past ten years. Thank you.

Toni, you gorgeous loving spirit, who taught me about humility amid all the chaos, and always has time to listen, especially after I have attended a birth – thank you, thank you, thank you.

Midwife/doula friend Faye, mother of four, who still gives me her full attention and support in a loving and caring way, amid all of her chaos. You are an angel.

My friend and confidante Nat, with the beautiful soul that sings. From our first conceptions we were drawn together as friends for life. It has truly been an honour to know you and to share our three pregnancies together. Thank you for the friendship we have.

Sue who has been a constant presence in my life, and now in my daughter's life. I cannot express in words what I have gained from our friendship. You have strength of character, and a Midas touch for everything you throw your heart into. Thank you for showing Jaeosha and I that anything is possible, because it really is possible. Nat the under water sea nymph, and twin soul sister, who taught me how to laugh at myself and the world again with our twisted sense of humor. I thank you for the friendship and support that we give each other.

My beautiful children, Jaeosha, Ben and Jarrad who came into this world in the most peaceful way. I love you all with all my heart and could not imagine my life without each and every one of you. Thank you for teaching me so many of the lessons of life that I need to learn. May your lives be happy, peaceful and full of love. I wish you enough – always. Believe in yourselves.

A special thankyou to Leigh Dick-Read, step-son of Dr Grantly Dick-Read, who has given me his blessings to use his step-father's work in this book. Leigh has to be the most passionate and enthusiastic male that I know when it comes to talking about natural birth. Thank you for your enthusiasm, support and humour.

And lastly, a BIG thankyou to Mary Murphy my wonderful midwife, who made my three waterbirth experiences brilliant and possible. You taught me that patience is a virtue – when I was over being pregnant, and great things come to those who wait. Thank you for believing in me and teaching me so much about labour and birth through my own and others experiences.

Notes

1. Dick-Read, G., *Childbirth Without Fear*, Pinter Martin, London, 1963: page 77.

2. ibid. page 89.

3. & 4. Wang, E. and Smaill, F., 'Infection in pregnancy', in Chalmers, I., Enkin, M., Keirse, Marc J.N.C. (eds); Effective Care in Pregnancy and Childbirth (2nd edition), Oxford University Press, Oxford, New York, 1989: page 123.

5. Hunter, D. and Keirse, Marc J.N.C., 'Gestational diabetes', in Enkin, M., Keirse, M., Renfrew, M., & Neilson, J, A Guide to Effective Care in Pregnancy and Childbirth (2nd edition), Oxford University Press, Oxford, New York, 1996: page 57.

6. ibid. page 58.

7. Gaskin, Ina May, *Ina May's Guide to Childbirth*, Bantam, New York, 2003: page 147.

8. Buckley, S., 'Ecstatic Birth: The Hormonal Blueprint for Labour', Mothering, March/April 2002.

9. England, P. & Horowitz, R., *Birthing from Within*, Partera Press, New Mexico, 1998: page 197

10. Gaskin, Ina May, *Ina May's Guide to Childbirth*, Bantam, New York, 2003: page 148.

11. Buckley, S., 'Ecstatic Birth: The Hormonal Blueprint for Labour', Mothering, March/April 2002.

12. ibid.

13. Gaskin, Ina May, *Ina May's Guide to Childbirth*, Bantam, New York, 2003: page 170.

14. England, P. & Horowitz, R., *Birthing from Within*, Partera Press, New Mexico, 1998: page 134.

15. Dick-Read, G., *Childbirth Without Fear*, Pinter & Martin, London, 1963: page 173.

16. Gaskin, Ina May, *Ina May's Guide to Childbirth*, Bantam, New York, 2003: page 165.

17. Balaskas, J. & Gordon, J., *Water Birth*: The Concise Guide to Water for Pregnancy, Birth and Infancy, Unwin Hyman, London, 1990: page 3.

18. Gaskin, Ina May, *Ina May's Guide to Childbirth*, Bantam, New York, 2003: page 174.

19. ibid: page 136.

20. Dick-Read, G., *Childbirth Without Fear*, Pinter & Martin, London, 1963: page 76.

21. ibid: page 75.

22. Gaskin, Ina May, *Ina May's Guide to Childbirth*, Bantam, New York, 2003: page 179.

23. Kitzinger, S., The New Pregnancy and Childbirth, Doubleday, New York, 1992: page 245.

24. & 25. Gaskin, Ina May, *Ina May's Guide to Childbirth*, Bantam, New York, 2003: page 158.

26. Noble, E., Childbirth With Insight, Houghton Mifflin, London, 1984: page 65.

27. Kitzinger, S., The New Pregnancy and Childbirth, Doubleday, New York, 1992: page 296.

28. & 29. Gaskin, Ina May, *Ina May's Guide to Childbirth*, Bantam, New York, 2003: page 245.

30. Dick-Read, G., *Childbirth Without Fear*, Pinter Martin, London, 1963: page 76.

31. Gaskin, Ina May, *Ina May's Guide to Childbirth*, Bantam, New York, 2003: page 258.

32. Kitzinger, S., *Breastfeeding Your Baby*, Doubleday, New York, 1998: page 18.

33. Field, M., 'Placentophagy', Midwives Chronicles & Nursing Notes, 1984.

34. ibid.

35. ibid.

36. Kitzinger, S., *Breastfeeding Your Baby*, Doubleday, New York, 1998: page 18.

37. ibid: page 44.

References

- Balaskas, J. & Gordon, J., *Water Birth*: The Concise Guide to Water for Pregnancy, Birth and Infancy, Unwin Hyman Limited, London, 1990.
- Buckley, S., 'Ecstatic Birth: The Hormonal Blueprint for Labour', Mothering, March/April 2002.
- Cole, B., Mummy Laid An Egg!, Red Fox (www.randomhouse.co.uk). Diamont, A., *The Red Tent*, St Martin's Press, 1998.
- Dick-Read, G., *Childbirth Without Fear*, Pinter & Martin, London, 1963 (revised edn 2005).
- England, P. & Horowitz, R., *Birthing from Within*, Partera Press, New Mexico, 1998.
- Enkin, M., Keirse, Marc J.N.C. (eds); Effective Care in Pregnancy and Childbirth (2nd edition), Oxford University Press, Oxford, New York, 1989. (3rd edn 2000).
- Field, M., 'Placentophagy', Midwives Chronicles & Nursing Notes, 1984.
- Gaskin, Ina May, *Ina May's Guide to Childbirth*, Bantam, New York, 2003.
- Gillespie, C., Your Pregnancy Month by Month, Harperpaperbacks, New York, (5th edn), 1998.
- Hodnett, E. D., 'Continuity of care givers for care during pregnancy and childbirth', The Cochrane Database of Systematic Reviews, 1998, Issue 3, 2005.

- Kitzinger, S., *Breastfeeding Your Baby*, Doubleday, New York, 1998. Kitzinger, S., The New Pregnancy and Childbirth, Doubleday, New York, 1992. See also, Dorling Kindersley edition, 2003.
- Mongan, M., HypnoBirthing: The Mongan Method: A natural approach to a safe, easier, more comfortable birthing, Rivertree Publishing, Concord, New Hampshire, (3rd edn), 2005.
- Noble, E., Childbirth With Insight, Houghton Mifflin, London, 1984.
- Odent, M., *The Scientification of Love*, Free Association Books, London, 1999.

Index

A

abdominal bracing 90
acupuncture 315
adrenalin 289
affirmations 134
aginal birth after a previous Caesarean (VBAC) 313
Andrea Robertson 217
anterior lip 212
antibiotics 277
anus 259
aquatic exercise classes 45
Australian Bush Flower Emergency Essence 63

B

baby swim 19
Bach Flower Rescue Remedy 63
bath 67
beanbag 64
beliefs about birth 52
birth-day 59
birth hormones 140
Birth hormones 268
birthing centre 12, 58
birthing position 219
birthing tub 207
birth plan 170
birthright 52
bladder 199
blood glucose levels 204
bloody show 189
bonding 41
Braxton Hicks 189
breastfeeding 227
Breaststroke 85
breathing 108
breech birth 313

C

cabbage leaves 245
caesarean 261
calming 133

care provider 51
cascade of intervention 53
castor oil 185
catecholamines 192
Charkovsky 321
childbirth education 6
Chinese Burn' 224
choices 177
chronic reflux 260
coach 286
community midwifery program 56
conception 51
continuity of care 59
contractions 136
cord clamping 232, 233
C-section 265
CTG machine 163
cycle 153

D

Dick-Read 8
dilation 37
disempowering 47
dolphins 43
dorsal horn 144
doula 153

E

ecstatic 313
EDD 288
Emergency Essence 146
endorphins 78, 311
England 295
engorgement 244
episiotomy 275
established labour 281
Estelle Myers 322
estimated date 101
exercise 299
exercises 300
expressed milk 283

F

Failure to progress 111

family bed 248
Family Birthing Centre 272
fear 11
Fear-Tension-Pain Syndrome 124
first trimester 60
fitball 63
foetal monitoring 64
Food 64

G

Gaskin 113
Gate Theory 144
genitals 35
Gestational Diabetes 261
glucose 261
glucose tolerance test 261

H

head moving 79
homebirth 184
homeopathic remedies 185
hormones 193
hospital 193
hospital policies 59
hot packs 196
hydrotherapy 81
hyper-extending 45
HypnoBirthing 152

I

Igor 321
Ina May Gaskin 113
independent childbirth education 6
induction 14, 283
intensity 161
internal examination 112
intervention 161

K

Kitzinger 214

L

labour 214

Labour Hormones 9
labour space 140
lactation consultant 239
land- based aerobic classes 89
listeria 257
love-making 89

M

massage 85
mastitis 245
medical specialist 53
meditation 144
membranes 189
mental preparation 290
Michel Odent 50
midwife 291
Midwifery care 56
monitoring 55
morning sickness 295
Mothering 326
music 133

N

natural birth 14
natural opiates 41
natural pain relief 65
nesting 121
nipple puller 242
Nipple stimulation 185
nitrous oxide 158
noises 289
nurturing environment 44

O

Obstetric Care 51
obstetrician 52
orgasm 116
orgasmic birth 214
orgasmic experience 116
overdue 118
ow glycemic index (GI) foods 77
oxytocin 109

P

pain relief 111
pain threshold 56
Pam 137
Pam England 37
Parenting 76
parturition 138
passively active 134
pelvic examination 199
pelvic-floor exercises 93
pelvic-floor muscles 92
pelvic opening 217
pelvis 218
performance anxiety 210
perineal massage 223
perineal preparation 221
perineum 218
period pain 292
pethidine 302
philosophy 21
piggyback contractions 208
placenta 231
placentophagy 234
planning 239
PNF stretching 300
poo 301
positions 135
post natal depression 235
pregnancy aquatic exercise classes 45
pregnancy resource centre 57
Prostaglandins 109
pubic bone 218
public hospital 58
pushing 77

R

reflexology 266
reflux 260
relaxation 81
relaxin 85
Rescue Remedy 146
Rhythmical Breathing 147
rupture of the membranes 258

S

sacroiliac joint 137
Scented oils 146
sciatica 85
second stage 202
sex 214
shared-care 59
Sheila Kitzinger 214
siblings 64
skin to skin 229
sleeping 249
sphincter 260
Strep B 260
subconscious mind 37
sucking reflex 140
suckle 41
surrendering 37
sweating 29
swimming 24
synthetic prostaglandin 118

T

tearing 117
TENS (Transcutaneous Electrical Nerve Stimulation) machine 144
testicles 35
The Five-Minute Time-Out Rule 170
Thoracic kyphosis 91
transition 78
tub 160

U

umbilical cord 273
urge to push 285
uterine muscles 78
uterus 87

V

vacuum extraction 291
vagina 293
vaginal examination 161
Valsalva Manoeuver, 220
VBAC 313
Vernix 66

W

walking 228
water 222
weight distribution 45
whales 19
wheat bags 144

Y

yoga 275

www.ingramcontent.com/pod-product-compliance
Lightning Source LLC
Chambersburg PA
CBHW060148050426
42446CB00013B/2720